What others have to say about Ch

"Brilliant!!! Read this simple and easy to understand book for practical ideas any person can use to propel their health, their appearance and their energy level while getting an inside peak at how celebrities, athletes and normal folk achieve amazing results!"

Mark Victor Hansen
Co-creator, *New York Times* best-selling series *Chicken Soup for the Soul®*
Co-author, *The One Minute Millionaire*

"If you're looking for a no-nonsense, state-of-the-art approach to weight loss and fitness, then get a copy of Christopher Guerriero's book, *Maximize Your Metabolism.* This is a book that separates fact from fiction and covers every important lifestyle, physiological and psychological issue in depth—and in a way that will get you more motivated than you have ever been. If you follow Christopher's program, you will succeed and develop the healthy attractive body that you want."

Lloyd Glauberman, Ph.D.
President, Psycho-Technology, Inc.
Developer of Hypno-Peripheral Processing

". . . 192 lbs fat to 135 lbs thin in 97 days! Thanks Christopher"

Jennifer Millner
Homemaker and mother of two
Age 54

"After 40 years of in-depth research studying with some of the greatest teachers in the world, I have to say that Christopher's material is the most complete work I have come across. Anyone following his direction would not only understand the meaning of Holistic [health & fitness] Success, they would experience dramatic improvements in all areas of their life. I want to personally congratulate him and I will definitely recommend it to all of my students worldwide."

Bob Proctor
Chairman, Life Success Institute
Author of the best-selling book *You Were Born Rich*

"This incredible book changed (saved) my life. It will be my gift to everyone I know for years to come."

Sandy Watkinson
Real Estate Professional

"Often books either touch on the 'How-To's' of personal fitness or personal growth. *Maximize Your Metabolism* does both in an unique and valuable way. In today's fast-paced world, this book gives an innovative approach to increased energy—FAST!"

Vince Poscente
Olympic Athlete
Speed Skiing Record holder – 135 mph
Author, *Invinceable Principles*

"Christopher Guerriero's holistic mind, body, spirit approach to fitness is clearly state of the art. No one has combined the art and science of personal health in one, easy to follow 'how to' book. Guerriero is the guru for fitness in the new millennium!"

Tim Ciasulli
2 Time National and World Offshore Powerboat Racing Champion
4 Time World Speed Record Holder

"Christopher's techniques are great! They are the most up to date I have ever found. I use them to help reach my personal goals. I also use that same knowledge to help my own clients reach their goals. I suggest that anyone who wants to cut thru all the gimmick diets and cut years off their efforts to make use of this information."

Kevin Beegle, C.P.T., P.R.C.S., Y.F.I., H.F.I., A.F.I.
Personal Fitness Trainer – 9 years

"I've never written a testimonial for anyone in the past, and I doubt I will ever be compelled to write one again, but reading this book was the best investment that I've made in years. I suggest anyone wanting to better their health and their physique read it and put it to good use—if you do, you'll be so far ahead of where you are right now that people will be asking you to help them get a body just like yours."

Michael Maas, Jr.
Personal Trainer – 12 years

"I can't thank you enough for helping me formulate a new diet and training program that worked! I just got my blood test back and my cholesterol dropped from 265 to 185. As you know, I had tried changing my diet before but was not able to make a significant impact. I'm glad I consulted with you before I let my doctor increase my cholesterol medication. On top of reaching that goal I was able to lose 15 pounds (by eating more food!). Thanks again for helping me achieve my goals. I could not have done it without your help."

John Watson
President, Premium Color Graphics, Inc.

"I lost 54 pounds in 6 weeks! People give me compliments everywhere I go. The techniques in this book just work, plain and simple."

Marilyn Gersham
Mother of 3

"It certainly is an honor to write about how Christopher's techniques have changed my life. When I first started using Christopher's system I was a size 12 and totally out of shape. My energy level was low and so was my level of concentration. We started our training routine, meeting 3 times a week, and gradually incorporated dietary changes. After a few weeks I noticed a difference in all aspects of my daily life. I felt younger, had a great deal more energy and stamina AND most significantly my clothing size just kept getting smaller and smaller. Chris' diet, as far as I was concerned, was a 'no brainer.' I was eating more food now than I had when I wasn't on a diet. My body was no longer that of a 54 year old and my outlook on life was that NOTHING was too difficult. I went down to a size 2 and all those people who said I was just 'big-boned' are still in shock at how good I look. The most amazing thing is Chris' approach to exercise. He takes the most difficult exercises, breaks them down into small, simple, non-threatening steps and before you know it you've accomplished some pretty advanced and amazing things. One wonderful thing about Chris is that he NEVER lets you languish in your success. He will always say 'Now when you do this exercise let's just make this one little change. . . .' That one simple little change brings the exercise to a new level and you're on your way to a new plateau."

Karen Horwitz
Real Estate Broker
Wife and Mother of 3

"Using the techniques outlined in this book unrealistic gains became achievable. I managed to quickly shed unwanted fat while increasing lean muscle. These techniques truly work!"

Kenneth Cop
Police Officer
Age 28

"This diet and fitness plan is absolutely amazing! No other program I had ever tried in the past was able to deliver on the results it promised so quickly, and I've tried them all. In only 30 days I lost 10 pounds and was in total disbelief as I watched my workout poundages actually increase! This program is a complete blueprint to being healthy and feeling great for a lifetime!"

Dave Wohlman
Senior Account Executive
Age 38

"Christopher Guerriero is the patron saint of internal fitness. When I began searching for the best to learn from, I was told that Christopher was the ONLY one to talk with—he's inspiring, insightful and incredibly knowledgeable."

Theresa Lynch
Business Owner
Age 29

"I have always been into staying in shape and keeping a healthy life style by working out, eating right, and using supplements to fill in my nutritional gap. Thanks to the techniques laid out in this book, I have learned so much more about fitness and nutrition. By following these principles, I have been able to drop more body fat and increase my energy level, as well as maximizing my metabolism."

Martin J. Michalski, M.S., C.P.A.
Senior Accountant
Age 27

"I've used these special techniques for approximately five years now. They help me become healthier, stronger and most importantly they helped to build the endurance within my joints—now I'm back to playing tennis, skiing and golfing. Follow this program and I'm confident you'll experience the same great results."

Paul Horwitz
Certified Public Accountant

"I received a copy of this book in the mail early this morning, I began reading it and was unable to put it down until I had finished many hours later. The detail and the uniqueness of Christopher's approach to helping people amazed me. This book is ahead of its time. Although it was late when I finished reading it, I went to my computer and composed a heartfelt thank you to Christopher and an email to all of my personal clients telling them that this book is mandatory reading."

Chuck Sanders, C.P.T.
Personal Trainer – 5 years

"I've read them all, but none have actually offered me the amount of knowledge and the motivation that *Maximize Your Metabolism* does. My shelves are lined with nutrition and fitness books, but this book is the only one I actually keep on my desk and refer to regularly."

Cynthia Bergman, C.P.T.
Personal Trainer – 13 years

Maximize Your Metabolism

Double your Metabolism in 30 Days or Less!

CHRISTOPHER V. GUERRIERO

This book is dedicated to my dear Patricia,
one of the most beautiful inspirations in my life
and a never-ending source of help and dedication
to all of my pursuits.

Notice: *Maximize Your Metabolism* is not intended as a substitute for the medical recommendations of physicians. This book is sold with the understanding that neither the author nor publisher is engaged in directly or indirectly dispensing medical advice or prescribing treatment for any kind of disease.

The intent is to offer information to help you, the reader, cooperate with other health and fitness professionals in your mutual quest for optimum weight loss, fitness, and good health. Since every person's metabolic response and general health requirements will differ, it is strongly emphasized that any person desiring to use this program, or any other dietary, fitness, or health program, should consult first with his or her doctor and should remain under the doctor's close medical supervision and advice. The information and ideas in this book are for educational purposes and are not intended as prescriptive advice. Consult your physician before starting any exercise or weight-loss program.

Acknowledgments

It has taken me a lifetime to acquire the knowledge that I am about to share with you, and throughout that lifetime I have been surrounded by the best of people. As I begin to reflect on the magnitude of this project and the profound impact it has had on so many, I am reminded of those who were instrumental in its development.

First and foremost, I wish to express my heartfelt thanks to Patricia for keeping me well fed each morning as I wrote and rewrote the contents of this book.

I would also like to thank my parents and my entire family for their love, a love that has helped ground and strengthen me throughout the years.

Among my greatest sources of inspiration are my clients, who have provided the impetus for my passion about life and living. Their desire to keep getting healthier, stronger, and better looking fuels my creativity. Together, we have worked miracles, and for this I thank them wholeheartedly.

I also wish to salute all the experts, teachers, mentors, and motivators who have shaped my life, my philosophies, my strategies, and my skills.

Finally, I would like to express my gratitude to you, the reader, with whom I feel a special bond because you are just getting started on your journey to a higher state of fitness. Although you cannot yet see the results in your physical appearance, I know that over the next few weeks—as you digest what this book has to offer—all of your dreams will come true.

You are all responsible in some way for this book. I thank all of you, and I wish you all the health, wealth, and happiness you desire in life.

Contents

Preface

My university studies in nutrition have been both a blessing and a bane. Those years of schooling taught me much about the process of nourishing the human body. However, I also discovered that the more formal education one has on "good nutrition," the *less* one actually knows about how to help people reach their health and fitness goals.

The problem, of course, is the considerable time lag between academic discovery and meaningful application. By the time things get studied by scientists, then categorized and studied again, written about in textbooks, and delivered to the universities to be studied by the next generation, the information is already out of date!

In all this there is a blessing, however. The science of nutrition and exercise—and the way they both affect the human body—changes almost as rapidly as the computer industry. (For the reader who is not familiar with the computer industry, it practically doubles every year.)

What does all this mean? Well, for one thing, it means that the most up-to-date individuals in the field of nutrition and fitness are not necessarily the most highly "schooled." Rather, the real experts are the ones who are in the field, testing each of the new theories, reading books, going to seminars, listening to tapes, and experimenting with all that seems viable. They then adopt the most valuable aspects of each theory or approach and discard the rubbish that inevitably finds its way in. And that's what I've done here. This book is a culmination of over fifteen years of research, trial and error, and experimentation to find the techniques that **guarantee great results**—and do so *every time they are properly used.*

There are really only three ways to proceed in choosing a nutrition and fitness regimen:

- Spend years reading, learning, and doing your own experiments (way too time consuming for most folks)
- Follow the crowd (not very wise, since the crowd is what keeps getting fatter and less healthy each year)
- Follow proven paths that have been developed from years of practical experiments

It is precisely for the benefit of those who choose the third option that this book was written.

I've spent years studying people who have successfully mastered their metabolism. I wanted to know what set them apart from the rest—and exactly what it was that they did that made them so successful—while their neighbors failed to obtain comparable results, regardless of how hard they seemed to diet and exercise.

I was driven by the notion that millions of people would benefit from this information if it could be distilled into a practical, easy-to-follow guide that *systematized* the **secrets for success**. When I use the term *secrets* here, I simply mean the tactics that only the few successful people were regularly using, the same tactics that the unsuccessful people seem to consistently skip over. Since no one else had stepped forward and done this, I decided to put all my expertise down on paper—and to finally share the truth about how to instantly and permanently stimulate your metabolism.

The system that follows represents the fruits of these many years of research and testing. It's the culmination of a long-term, multidisciplinary research project to create an easy-to-understand, personal guide to mastering your metabolism. My goal in creating this book is to help you master yours.

The World Has Been Waiting

As you might expect, virtually all health and exercise programs are crammed to the rafters with clients who are desperate to gain the upper hand on their metabolism so they can lose unwanted pounds and regain their youthful figures.

Many of these men and women have unfortunately been suckered into the whirlwind of diets, gadgets, and weight-loss theories that invariably promise far more than they deliver. They're victims of the false marketing and ridiculous claims of the diet and exercise industries that have been brainwashing us for years.

They've tried to lose weight with every plan imaginable. They've read books, listened to tapes, even joined groups. Perhaps once or twice in their dieting lives, they've caught a fleeting glimpse of their ideal weight, but they've *never achieved their ideal on a sustained basis.* Within a few months or a year, their weight had invariably zoomed right back to a disappointingly high level.

These are the overweight men and women who are regularly beating a path to the doors of health clubs, mine included, only to find that their goal of permanent weight loss is as elusive as the calorie-free hot-fudge malt. The difference between what other clubs do and what my health clubs have done (and what you'll learn about in this book) is that we take a whole-body approach to health. We help our clients master their metabolism by using a systematic process, and it is that systematic process that's laid out in detail in this book.

My Search for the Answer

It was the desperate longing for an effective weight-loss regimen on the part of all these fitness seekers that inspired me in the late 1980s to launch my search for the perfect metabolic enhancers. At that time, early clinical research was making important new discoveries which hinted that metabolic rate is not the intractable biological enemy of the overweight. In other words, it was found that one's metabolism is not necessarily predetermined by genetics. Rather, metabolism is an aspect of one's physiology that is amenable to dramatic change—indeed, a change that can be realized in a relatively short period of time.

The secret that was unfolding, ever so slowly, was that introducing certain dietary nutrients into the body at key times during the day—into the body of a person with the proper physical and mental training, that is—can (and does!) induce the metabolic rate to rise, thereby literally turning the human body into a fat-burning furnace with a voracious appetite for melting unwanted fat.

In other words, *if you know how to do it*, it is possible to speed up your metabolism and lose unwanted weight, permanently. And the *how* turns out to be a formula which is so scientific that it could be duplicated in almost any individual who's willing to make certain changes in the way they live.

It's that formula that I was striving to come up with, and through years of research I found it! I discovered that the secret to losing weight is not to be found merely in trying new diets or new weight-loss programs. Only when you *change your metabolism* will you finally vanquish your enemy and free yourself from the dieting roller coaster.

To create a program that could readily be duplicated by all who used it presented special difficulties. After all, we're all different and our metabolisms ebb and flow at different rates. Moreover, I wanted a program that was all encompassing, one that included every factor that could have a profound, healthful effect on a person's metabolism.

To achieve that goal, I traced all the elements of the successful programs that were out there and I tossed out all the fluff. Then an amazing thing happened: Once there were only a few elements left on the drawing board, it finally all made sense. I realized that the "active ingredients" of various individual approaches were capable of working in concert to boost human metabolism, almost forcing a slow metabolism to rise—indeed, to *far surpass its normal level.*

That discovery is the main reason why I have made education the cornerstone of the mission and operational strategy of each of the companies I have established. I believe that once people learn how to develop their health, their fitness, and their metabolism, and once they invest in themselves and experience the amazing rewards, all the requisite ingredients for achieving success in life—motivation, confidence, and enthusiasm—will just naturally follow.

In all of my businesses, my staff and I strive to make continuing education an easy, inspiring part of every client's experience with us. If you haven't already visited one of my facilities, I invite you to do so; I believe it will change the way you think about fitness and nutrition. If you haven't had a chance to subscribe to one of my health and fitness newsletters or visited my Web site, I urge you to do that, too. Be sure to keep back issues of the newsletters on hand and make them part of your health and fitness library. Even if you read only a little at a time, you'll soon know more than most people ever will about what really makes our bodies work.

I hope you enjoy this book as much as I have enjoyed writing it for you.

Christopher V. Guerriero

****

I welcome interaction with my readers. You may contact me by e-mail, or postal mail.

Web site: **www.MaximizeYourMetabolism.com**
e-mail: **Author@MaximizeYourMetabolism.com**

Christopher V. Guerriero
In care of:
Wisdom Books, LLC.
292 Route 22 west
Green Brook, NJ 08812

This book was written with the sole objective of helping the reader achieve a stronger metabolism, better overall health, more energy, freedom from slow-working diets, and a more worthwhile life. Welcome to the newest technology of health and fitness management . . .

1

Prelude to the System

"There are two types of people in this world:
those who make their body fit their lifestyle
and those who make their lifestyle fit their body.
It's up to you to choose
which of these two categories you want to be in."

—Christopher V. Guerriero

We all have dreams of what we want to look like. We all want to believe deep down in our souls that we can and will look and feel great. We all want to be complimented on our looks and our physique, and even approached by others for advice on issues of health. For many of us, however, those dreams have largely taken second place to our day-to-day frustrations, to the extent that we no longer even make an effort to realize our dreams.

Before we go any further, I want to congratulate you, because by reading this book you have chosen to join the ranks of that top 10 percent of the population that will truly create their own physical destiny, rather than allowing their destiny to be determined by their current physical structure.

As you read this book during the next few days or weeks, you will grow and learn more than you could ever imagine. Just open your mind, forget everything you once thought to be set in stone, and enjoy the results.

Knowing how to achieve a state of true balance among the various parts of your body is the only way to embark on a health- and metabolism-enhancing diet. You need to know which areas inside your complex digestive system are working at optimum performance and which ones need to be rejuvenated.

Picture a table with only one leg. Even if you take the corner that's opposite that leg and lean it against a wall to get it to stand up, how likely is it to remain standing when you begin to place objects on top of it? Not likely at all. Now if that same table had two legs, it would probably last a bit longer. Three legs, even longer yet. And if the table had all four legs, I bet you could pile a whole bunch of stuff on top of it without disturbing the table's balance.

The same is true of your digestive and metabolic system. If there are any unbalanced hormonal, glandular, or nutrient reservoirs, a diet will produce results that are, at best, temporary and insignificant. Yet if you could remedy these imbalances as part and parcel of a dieting regimen, the results would not only be more healthful but also much more dramatic. The most powerful aspect of this book is that it holds the secrets to finally attaining balance within your body, but only if you combine all the techniques you encounter in it. As you make your way through the book, take your time and thoroughly read and implement the steps given in each chapter before going on to the next.

You will likely be surprised by the changes your body will make along the way. Finishing this book will become an adventure for you. One suggestion I usually give my personal clients is to take a photo of themselves before they start reading and implementing this program, and then take another photo, holding this book up, after they have completed it. Send me those photos for my files, and I'll more than likely use many of them in upcoming printings.

The Cardinal Rule of Losing Weight

Everyone knows how to lose weight and stay thin. All you have to do is burn more calories than you consume, right? Well, it's not quite that simple, but there is a very scientific way of handling this challenge that virtually guarantees results for everyone who follows the same formula. And that formula is what this book is all about. By the time you have made your way through it and implemented all the steps that are set forth along the way, you will have *Maximized Your Metabolism.*

The basis of permanent weight loss has never really changed: consume fewer calories and, at the same time, try to burn additional calories by moving your body to a greater degree than you were accustomed to moving it in the past. Unfortunately, the ability of humans to master this approach hasn't changed a whole lot, despite years of trying.

The result? Millions of Americans are locked in an endless struggle to control their weight and master their health. The trouble is that lurking behind the simplicity of the cardinal rule of weight loss is a problem of far greater difficulty. You may have heard it verbalized like this:

"I just can't seem to lose weight predictably."

"I think I've screwed up my metabolism."

"Professional" dieters, defined here as people who have dieted so many times they can't count them all, resoundingly report that repeated dieting causes major roadblocks to their efforts to lose weight and stay thin. Study after study has shown that the "yo-yo" dieting effect that we in America seem to be caught up in is very taxing to the correct functioning of our metabolism. Hence, our metabolic rate becomes slower and slower with each weight-loss–weight-gain cycle.

But that's not the only reason why our metabolisms may be a bit sluggish. The strength, or the "speed," of our metabolism is usually determined by several factors, such as

- Past dieting, especially attempts at rapid weight loss
- Age

  As a matter of fact, your metabolism begins to slow in early adulthood, at a rate of 2 percent per decade.
- Activity level

  Less active people generally have a slower metabolism.
- Lack of *proper* physical activity

  Certain exercises tend to increase a person's metabolism while others have only a slight effect on it. By making small but appropriate changes to your current level of activity, you could boost your metabolism massively (more on this in the chapter on exercise).
- Lack of proper meal placement during the day—every day

  One notion about weight loss that's prevalent in this country is that people can lose weight by skipping breakfast. Nothing could be further from the truth! In fact, eating a healthful breakfast actually *turns up* our fat-burning furnace (our metabolism) and gives us far more mental and physical energy for the first half of the day. A full description of how and when to eat for best results will be laid out for you later in this book.

Now let's get back to your past dieting attempts. Just look at the results and note the undesirable changes that seem to occur the *more times* you've dieted. By better than a two-to-one margin over less-frequent dieters, "professional" dieters have found that:

- Weight-loss strategies that used to be effective for them are showing far fewer results now
- Gaining weight has become easier
- Losing weight has become harder
- Dieting plateaus have become more frequent
- Weight loss is becoming increasingly hopeless

The cause of all of these common complaints is the slowing of your metabolism. Well, now is the time to put an end to that. Now is the time to take control of your metabolism—and your life. Now is the time to master your metabolism by following the course laid out in the following chapters. But be warned! Each chapter contains one step that will increase your metabolic rate and improve your health. Skipping one or more of these chapters may stop the process in its tracks. Very few people are aware of their own "weak link," the reason that their particular metabolism is not working at peak efficiency. Everyone who has attempted to lose weight through dieting has created one or more personal "weak links," and these weak links are the reason why other weight-loss programs fail to get you the results you want.

Each of the chapters in this book has been designed to *Maximize Your Metabolism* while minimizing each of your weak links. Every factor that affects your particular metabolism will become stronger and help boost your metabolic rate. If you find that you're tempted to skip one or more chapters, may I suggest that the techniques outlined in those chapters are probably the ones that your particular body needs the most.

Remember, you're seeking a new level of understanding of how your metabolism works, and at the same time you're training your metabolism to function at its optimum level.

Many overweight men and women find that trying to control their metabolic rate is nothing short of a hellish nightmare, and that's why the word "permanent" has never been part of their weight-loss vocabulary. One recent national survey showed, for example, that 66 percent of Americans were overweight. Translated into absolute numbers, this means that at least 90 million adults take in more calories than they burn up. Another review, this one called the National Health and Nutrition Examination Survey, showed that the number of overweight Americans increased by 8 percent between 1976 and 1988, and I'm willing to bet that the number has continued to increase in the years since 1988.

The sad thing is that not only are the overweight becoming *more numerous*, they're also getting *fatter*, despite the fact that there are more "weight-loss" products, creams, pills, and potions on the market today than ever before.

According to the National Center for Health Statistics, American men now weigh nearly 9 pounds more, on average, than in 1960, and American women weigh nearly 13 pounds more, on average, than their counterparts of just a *decade* ago.

How could this be possible? After all, in the past, people didn't know half of what they know today about proper diet and exercise! Just as one example, back in the 1960s there was a state-of-the-art exercise machine that I like to call the Fat Vibrator. You know what I'm talking about: the machine that had a large belt that a "fitness expert" would wrap around your waist. When the machine was turned on, the belt would "vibrate" the weight right off of your body. Well, this sounds funny to us now, but back then people really believed that it would help them lose weight—and there are versions of that machine still on the market today!

Yes, people are getting fatter, and, as a nation, we seem powerless to reverse this trend, despite our best attempts to do so. But the worst is almost surely yet to come: Though only about one in four Americans are obese, fully 80 percent of men and 70 percent of women over the age of forty are more than 10 pounds overweight. If you're in your twenties or thirties now and are having difficulty losing weight, you can well imagine how hard it will be for you to slim down in another ten or twenty years.

This book can end all that!

I don't profess to have uncovered, discovered, or developed anything new. I've simply spent more than a decade of my life studying various health-enhancing techniques, exercise regimens, nutritional programs, and more.

As a matter of fact, I've been so passionate about finding answers to the questions we've all had about how to permanently increase our body's ability to burn fat, get in shape, and stay healthy that at one point I was reading two books a week, attending seminars, and studying the effects of various weight-loss techniques by downloading information about them to my clients, who willingly took all this information and put it into practice for me.

The result is a proven set of strategies that will help you become leaner and healthier. This book gives you the principles you need to lose weight, fast!—without pain, without guilt, and, most importantly, without backsliding. The weight you lose will never, ever return, provided you make the modifications in your health and fitness regimen that are laid out in this text.

Sound too good to be true? Well, keep reading . . .

For over fifteen years now, I've been teaching men and women how to rev up their metabolism, lose weight, and become fit. I've personally witnessed their disappointment with weight-loss schemes that promise so much but deliver so little. By the time they get to me, they've been scammed by everything and everyone. They've tried the pills, the potions, the body wraps, and much more. They've joined local chapters of the big, national weight-loss chains. They've eaten those expensive, prepackaged meals. They've listened to the tapes that offer subliminal suggestions. They've read dozens of glittering magazine articles. And, of course, they've seen all the books in the bookstores. All this, and they're still looking for the answer. Well, here it is!

The Missing Link

What overweight people need, of course, is not another new diet. What is needed—but has never before been available—is a comprehensive program that shows you how to *Maximize Your Metabolism* effectively. That's the ultimate key to dealing with the weight-loss struggle, the *abracadabra* of opening up a whole new, magical way of healthful living.

This is what *Maximize Your Metabolism* promises, and this is what the techniques described herein will deliver.

Before I get down to the exciting details of why these techniques work and what they can do for *you*, I'm going to ask you to rethink many of the things you've been told about how to lose weight and stay thin.

Forget about losing weight the long, slow, "sensible" way

It is my opinion that the long, slow, moderate approach to permanent weight loss will never work for most overweight people. This business of bumping along, losing a pound this week and a half-pound the next through simple restriction in caloric intake, might work for a few iron-willed Victorians, but it will never work for the vast majority of people, simply because they just don't have the willpower or the time!

Don't get me wrong! I'm certainly not condoning or advocating rapid weight loss. On the contrary, the rate of weight reduction I'm recommending is not detrimental to good health, but it will show results faster than a pound a week, possibly far more.

It's important to keep in mind that the intent of this book is to improve your overall health and metabolism as well as your body's efficiency in utilizing the food you give it. Do not look upon it as just another "diet book," because that's neither what it is nor what it is meant to be. It was designed to give you a blueprint for attaining a higher metabolic rate in a healthful way. This blueprint will enable your body to burn up all the food you eat and to assimilate that food properly, so that your body utilizes all the nutrients in each mouthful of food and excretes all the waste that's produced in your day-to-day living.

The problem is that most overweight people have been on so many diets that they've made disturbing alterations to their metabolic systems. As a result, many of them are discovering that losing weight the old-fashioned, "sensible" way with 1200-calorie-per-day, low-fat diets just doesn't work anymore. Their weight loss comes to a halt, they get frustrated, and then they revert to their former pattern of overeating. Of course, the long, slow, sensible way does work for some overweight people. If it does, that's terrific. But in case it doesn't—and this is what happens more often than not—I'll teach you how to take the bull by the metabolic horns. I'll show you that losing weight a bit faster is not only the MOST sensible way to lose weight, but that for many overweight people it's the ONLY way to do so.

Forget about learning how to eat in "moderation"

Moderation is the straightest, surest road to mediocrity and weight-loss failure that has ever been invented. Now I know that most of the so-called weight-loss and behavior-modification experts preach the gospel of *moderation.* Nevertheless, I've learned through years of study that that doctrine is hopelessly inadequate and *rarely* produces the lasting change in behavior that you need.

To be sure, caloric restriction does have its merits, but not in maximizing your metabolic rate, and that's the focus of this book: raising your metabolism, keeping it high, and reaping all the benefits associated with that process.

Just tell me, for example, where all your attempts at moderation have gotten you. Well, if you're like most of the clients who come to my office, you've found that moderation was great for a short time; but then, with no prior notice, your results began to taper off dramatically, which is to say that your determination and effort were noticeably present but the fruits of your labor were not.

What's wrong, of course, is that while moderation may be a worthy path, it is far too flimsy a strategy to help you achieve your goal. In the case of long-term moderation, what occurs is a methodical *slowing* of your metabolism. As you cut down on your intake of food, you also cut down on your body's need to attain a high metabolic rate, and so your metabolism slows down. When you follow a moderation-type diet, you are in essence training your metabolism to work at a slower pace. Then, when you do eat or drink, that food or liquid can't be fully and efficiently digested, so it's stored . . . as fat!

Forget about denial

Just because you implement the strategies put forth in this book doesn't mean that you have to turn yourself into the type of person who can never enjoy a chocolate brownie or a dish of ice cream for fear of losing control. Successful metabolic control doesn't depend on long-term denial, and this powerful new program does not promote any such solution. Pumping up your metabolism is the name of the game, and it will turn you into a winner in no time at all.

Imagine the new freedom that comes with knowing that your revved-up metabolic system is always on duty, always ready, able, and eager to burn up those excess calories instead of turning them into fat as it once did. There's no denial here, just good, healthful living, making you fit and ready for action.

Forget what you've heard about exercise

In the course of my life, I've operated a successful nutritional consulting business and several large, upscale health clubs. Believe me, I've seen more than my share of misstatements and out-and-out lies made by an industry that sometimes seems more eager to help your billfold—not your body—to lose weight.

Contrary to what you've been told on those TV infomercials, exercise cannot turn you into a muscle-bound man or woman in six weeks or less. Exercise cannot transform fat into muscle. Exercise cannot cause "spot" reduction anywhere on your body. Moderate exercise cannot cause dramatic weight loss, no matter what they tell you.

Is exercise important to long-term weight control? You better believe it. But in this book, I'll show you that exercise's greatest contribution to weight control has less to do with the number of calories it induces your body to burn up than it does with the almost miraculous changes it makes in the way your metabolic system functions. Here's where the real payoffs come into play. If more Americans knew the full story of how exercise alters metabolic rate, the thought of embarking on an exercise program wouldn't be so scary—and a lot more than (the actual) 15 percent of adults would be exercising *regularly*.

In reality, exercise does burn off the calories that you consume, and if it's done properly it will also immediately burn off some of your stored fat. However, your actual motivation for exercising should be the increase in metabolic rate that will accrue from engaging in exercise on a regular basis. Even then, you won't significantly increase your metabolism unless you go about your exercise in the fashion that is explained in a later chapter of this book. This method will enable you to burn calories and body fat virtually all the time, even when you're not exercising, even when you're sleeping!

A promise to you . . .

Rebuilding your metabolic system and setting you up for lifelong health will take place in four orderly steps:

1. Cleansing your system
2. Reformulating your eating (times of meals, as well as quantity and quality of the food you consume)
3. Introducing strength-building and cardiovascular exercises into your life, to both stabilize and increase your metabolic rate for the long term
4. Training your mental core

Sound difficult? Believe me, it isn't. We've got plenty of great tips and motivational help to enable you to succeed in making these miraculous, life-enhancing changes. And the best part is that you can make them in thirty days or less! That's right! In less than the time between the dates of receipt of successive bank statements, you will have turned your system into a virtual furnace of metabolic activity that will have you losing weight, regaining good health, and carving out a richer, fitter future and a fuller life.

As mentioned earlier, each chapter contains a technique that will help you increase your metabolism, so you won't have to wait until you've completely finished this book before you begin to reap the rewards of the program. The book is laid out in such a way that you can read a chapter and then implement the strategy that's outlined there before moving on to the next chapter. But, please, do yourself a favor and stick with it; keep at the reading of the book until you've gotten all the way to the end. As a matter of fact, I recommend that you do yourself one better: go back and read it again.

More than a decade ago, I read that each time you read a book, you pick up something new—not because you missed it the first time through, but because you're not the same person you were when you read it the first time. Each time you read this book, you'll pick up new pieces to help you in the pursuit of your health and fitness goals. Each time you read this book—no, each time you reread each *chapter* (since you'll be implementing the techniques in each chapter as you go along)—you'll become a better, healthier person.

And There's More

Once you bring your metabolic rate under control, you will not, you simply *cannot*, believe the enormous difference it will make in bringing your weight under permanent control.

For many of my clients, the unwanted weight seemed to *automatically* disappear when their metabolic system took command of their dietary fat intake and used that fuel for power rather than for building up stores of fat. Believe me, you will be one powerful person! For the first time in your life, you'll be the one calling the shots, plus you'll get two additional benefits that are extremely worthwhile:

First, you'll be able to breeze through your culinary life unmindful of those years of eating taboos you've suffered through in years past. When you crank up your metabolic rate, you won't have to worry about those myriad do-I-or-don't-I eating situations that can turn an ordinary diet into disaster.

With this program, not only will your high-speed metabolic rate iron out the bumps and lumps in your road to a thinner you, but you'll also gain the upper hand in *how* you eat, *what* you eat, even *when* you eat. You'll have the power to "take it or leave it." If you want to enjoy an occasional sugary dessert, have a periodic nighttime snack, or even indulge in a rare caloric binge, you can do so, and yet your increased metabolic rate will save you from the weight volatility you've become so accustomed to.

Second—and this is perhaps the more important of the two benefits—this program launches you into a whole new orbit of better eating and better living, the physically fit way. That's right! You may have been missing out on huge parts of the good life because of your sluggish metabolism and your sedentary ways. No more! I want to give you the ability to be *content* with your every decision as to how, what, and when you eat, and I want you to feel good about those decisions, precisely *because* they are the decisions that you truly *wanted* to make. In other words, you won't feel guilty or ashamed every time you take a bite of food.

Eating is such a natural activity that you should feel great when you engage in it (before, during, and after). You simply must learn to eat the correct foods and to eat at the proper times. I believe that one of the greatest downfalls of all of the poorly designed dieting programs that are out there is that they make people feel bad about eating! After all, what's bad about eating? *Eating is what enables us to survive and to thrive.* You should keep in mind that it's only the act of making poor *choices* about what we eat that cuts down on how long we survive and whether we thrive.

I promise that by the time you've finished this four-course menu for self-change and empowerment, you'll be able to do both (survive *and* thrive). Finally, you'll start behaving around food in ways that so-called normal people do. You'll enjoy life as you've never enjoyed it before, without craving the junk food that may have been your downfall in the past!

> There are certain Universal Laws of health, and you'll learn some of the most important ones in this book. The concept of a Universal Law can easily be illustrated by a non–health-related law that you are no doubt familiar with: the Law of Gravity.
>
> The Law of Gravity, like all Universal Laws, was not made by humans. It says that if you jump off a cliff, you will fall down; you won't be propelled upwards or sideways. You may not even be aware of the law of gravity, but you will fall just the same. You may think the law of gravity is stupid, false, or unfair, and you may even argue the point; nevertheless, you will fall.
>
> The same is true of the Universal Laws of health: you may not actually believe that consuming adequate amounts of water will have a profound impact on your metabolism, your weight, your health, and your looks, but it has those effects all the same; in fact, it has a very profound effect, as do all the Universal Laws of health.

The Golden Road Ahead

The bottom line is this: the principles in this book will work, regardless of how long you've been overweight, how much weight you may need or want to lose, or how many times you've failed. Since this program is based on science, it can work for you. Just apply the easy techniques put forth in this book, and you'll develop unshakable self-control and stop your overeating behavior dead in its tracks.

With each powerful step of this program, you'll learn new, take-charge strategies to change the way you behave. Each day, you'll build on the success of the day before. In no time at all, you'll be a person who has control over your life and your weight. You'll be a person who's leaner, more attractive, and more energetic. And you'll be a person you can admire, a person who has won the respect and admiration of family and friends. I promise you that all of this will come about—you *will* be successful—if you simply follow the strategies laid out in this book.

I started my research with the actual dieting process, since this is the one aspect that the majority of my clients kept insisting that I help them with. Thus, I will begin here with a discussion of dieting, but before I do, please be advised that this is not a diet book and that I do not profess to be an expert in dieting. I know a few techniques that work for everyone who follows them (with few exceptions, such as people with intense medical challenges or physical limitations—and those people should definitely consult a physician prior to embarking on this program and request instructions as to how to alter it in order to meet their specific needs).

There are a few basics that need to be followed in dieting, including an initial cleansing routine that I will not go into now (though I will cover it in great detail later).

First, you must consume slightly less than your body expels throughout the day. Then you must cut out all the foods that limit your efficiency, such as sugars and sweets, added fats (including, but not limited to, all fried foods), alcohol, all drugs (except those prescribed by your physician), all processed foods, and all dairy products except egg whites (we'll get into this more in a later part of the book). Then you must further limit your intake of starchy foods, such as breads, pasta, potatoes, and beans. You do need to include in your diet some foods that are fresh, clean sources of protein, such as fish, chicken, and egg whites, and you need to eat some fresh, raw, colorful vegetables.

I know, I know! At this point you're thinking to yourself, "But you said that we weren't going to have to sacrifice the foods we wanted!" Now stop complaining! I'm not finished, and I never said that you could eat poorly and still be healthy. You must eat healthfully, exercise properly, and train your mind to help you in the process. Then you can eat your favorite foods on occasion without any negative consequences, because your metabolism will be so high that as soon as you eat that chocolate cake your metabolism will burn it right up. (Note that I said *on occasion*. You cannot do this sort of thing very frequently!)

Now that's the basics, and here's where it has brought me: after experimenting for months with my clients, I found that after they had done all of this, we could further manipulate their metabolism by introducing certain foods at specific times of the day. Yes, you may have heard of this before, things like eating your carbohydrates mostly in the morning and, as the day goes on, slowly increasing your intake of clean (low-fat) protein and decreasing your intake of carbohydrates. However, there's more to this part of the equation. We can combine certain foods at a single meal to help your body with the digestive process.

What does all this mean? It's simple. Now we have the basis for altering our metabolism as we see fit. Don't worry if you don't yet get it. I'm going to give you an example later, in the chapter on dieting.

After the dieting part of the equation was completed, I found that it was possible to duplicate these amazing results in client after successful client. Only then did I begin working on the fitness aspect of the program. Exercise is a key ingredient. If you're not convinced that exercise is vital to a healthful lifestyle, you need this chapter more than anyone else, so clear your mind and concentrate.

Different forms of exercise help us in different ways. Aerobic (cardiovascular type) exercise helps us by strengthening our heart muscle and by increasing the amount of oxygen in our bloodstream. Oxygen helps us burn fat and build strong muscles. Now *strong* muscles are not necessarily *large* muscles, so if you're like some of my clients who desperately want to avoid building muscles, don't worry! We're not here to build muscle size, but we do want to build muscle density, which not only makes us stronger and healthier but also builds both our immune system and our metabolism.

Note: If you would like to build large muscles, then check out my web site at **www.MaximizeYourMetabolism.com**. There's a special section there just for you.

The other form of exercise we'll be doing is *anaerobic*. For purposes of this book, we'll use that term to describe weight-bearing exercises. While aerobic exercise will allow us to burn body fat as we exercise and maybe even for a few hours afterwards, anaerobic exercise makes it possible for us to burn body fat *at all times* (even when we're sitting down or sleeping).

Now what I just said is quite well known and not too hard to understand, although we'll go into more detail on it in the chapter on exercise. But we're going to take this a step further. In a chapter dedicated to the all-so-important topic of anaerobic exercise, I'll show you a specific exercise routine that will tremendously increase your metabolism.

The final aspect of this metabolic equation that we've been discussing is mental training. Creating and holding an image of yourself as someone who has already achieved your goals is *mandatory* for fast and lasting success. I cannot be more convinced of this fact. This is the point that all other programs have mistakenly left out. Maybe they didn't know about its importance at the time, or maybe they thought you wouldn't believe that your mind could have such a profound impact on your health and your appearance. Believe it or not, what you focus on during the day is what determines your success. To emphasize this fact, I'll quote two pioneers in the field of mind development.

The popular success philosopher Napoleon Hill once wrote:

> Whatever the human mind can conceive and believe it can achieve.

According to William James, the eminent Harvard psychologist of the early 1900s:

> The greatest discovery of the nineteenth century was not in the realm of physical science, but the power of the subconscious (mind) touched by faith.

James concluded:

> Every individual can tap into an eternal reservoir of power that will enable them to [achieve] bodily healing, financial independence, spiritual awakening, prosperity beyond your wildest dreams.

The knowledge that we can alter our surroundings with our mind dates back centuries. And I'm not here to quote scripture, but the power of the mind is also noted in every major religious text, including the Bible:

Everything is possible for him who believes.

According to your faith will it be done to you.

Training the mind is at least as important in our process to rapidly reach our goals as exercise and dieting combined. A person can never outperform their own self-image, so implanting the right image in your mind from the start is vital—and it may take some time, since you've probably been walking around all these years with a poor image of yourself when it comes to your body.

I recently heard a story that vividly illustrates this point. A study was carried out to measure the correlation between the incidence of breast cancer in women in America and women's feelings toward their breasts. It's no wonder that this nation has both the highest breast-augmentation (enlargement) rate and the highest breast-cancer rate. If you hate a part of your body so much that you're willing to have surgery to alter it, that hate (whether it be conscious or subconscious) will cause problems for you internally.

What we'll be dealing with when you get to the chapter on mental training (the one entitled "Laser Visualization") is how to develop a positive self-image and a sense of passion about *how great you'll feel* once you've achieved your fitness goals.

Your mind is always the key to achieving your goals. Keeping your mind in a positive state as you progress through this program is paramount in achieving your physical goals.

In the chapter on visualization, you'll learn a technique for developing your inner image, which will then guide your outer results. In that chapter we'll discuss how to focus for thirty minutes each day on the person that you will become. You'll learn how to be detailed in your visualization and how to concentrate on every aspect of your life that will be improving: how other people will react to you, your new body, and your new energy level; what type of clothing you'll be wearing; what changes you'll be making in your hairstyle; etc.

Still More Testing

I continued to test and refine this system during countless hours with my clients. Slowly, the solution to the metabolic puzzle fell into place. What has gone into the making of this comprehensive, informative book you are now reading is the successful experience of tens of thousands of people who, like you, were seeking to improve their health, their appearance, and their metabolism. This included thousands of my personal clients, as well as members of my clubs who have worked with me or my staff.

An Avalanche of Interest

There are many people today who are following fat-loss and diet programs that are basically unhealthy. Most of these programs have no real emphasis on permanent fat loss or metabolic enhancement. Others can actually increase your susceptibility to potentially severe health problems. A properly planned fat-loss or metabolic-enhancement program should be specifically designed to improve your level of health as you achieve permanent fat loss through a heightened metabolism.

Many of us have potential hereditary problems: a family history of a certain disorder such as heart disease, high blood pressure, hypoglycemia, arthritis, or obesity. Often, a general diet plan that is good for one person can be very harmful to another. For example, a person with a family history of—and therefore a susceptibility to—heart disease should not be placed on a diet that can increase the risk of heart or circulatory problems, yet this practice is commonplace, especially with fad or gimmicky diet plans and programs.

The program that you are about to encounter was developed in the early 1980s after it was found that a person could significantly increase their metabolic rate by introducing certain nutrients into their system at specific points throughout the day. The program employs what I call the Pyramid System of caloric staggering. Put simply, a person follows three separate diets throughout the course of a week. Each of these diets provides a different level of calories, proteins, carbohydrates, fats, and fiber. I have found that adopting such a diet can and will greatly increase the rate at which a person's metabolism assimilates and distributes all of the nutrients taken in during the day.

In essence, this book was designed to provide you with the information and blueprints necessary for you to transcend your past limitations and go on to achieve massive results in every area of your physical well-being . . . and your life.

My mission in life thus far has been a simple one: to help as many people as possible to achieve their physical goals. I began by creating eating/dieting programs for those who wanted to achieve a healthier, more attractive appearance.

Because of the exacting nature of these programs, it took three business days to complete each diet for each individual client, which severely limited the number of clients I could work with. A few years after embarking on this endeavor, I came to the realization that I could help a lot more people if I simply trained others who could assist me in creating and disseminating these programs. And so it was that the challenge of teaching my techniques to others began.

The struggle became easier and easier as time went on, and I was fortunate to be working with people who were open-minded enough to test my program and read all the material I had developed up to that point. But I was still unable to offer help to *all* the people who contacted me. I then decided to open an office dedicated to creating an atmosphere that was conducive to helping my clients achieve their physical goals. Although this office eventually became a great health club, I still came to the nagging conclusion that I was limited to helping only the people who actually visited my clubs. It was becoming clear that the program had to be written down.

The development of these techniques has taken nearly fifteen years. During that time, the health field has changed immensely. In fact, as stated earlier, the health field changes on a weekly, if not daily, basis. Fad diets come and go, but so do the great schemes employed in the marketing of them. What remained after all the fads and gimmicks fell by the wayside were the golden laws that are contained in this book, the laws that govern every person's metabolism.

I hope you profit as much as all of my other clients have from this material. If you put yourself into it a hundred percent, I know you will.

Deep within man dwell those slumbering powers;
powers that would astonish him,
that he never dreamed of possessing;
forces that would revolutionize his life
if aroused and put into action.

—Orison Sweet Marden

One final note before we begin

I had to dig into both old and new scientific research to filter out science from science fiction for you, using a skeptical eye. This book provides you with a serious method of stepping up your metabolism. I realize the information that is contained herein is not for everyone. Some people will read this book and then put it right back on the shelf—or in the box that contains their other health, fitness, or dieting books. That's fine for them, but not for you. You've taken the first step by purchasing a book like this. You've proved that you want to learn and master your metabolism.

I hope you'll put this information to good use. It's taken me years to gather and condense this material into a workable system—a system of simple steps that will yield the results you seek, steps which have helped numerous personal clients of mine to achieve the goals they had set for themselves over the years.

Good luck, and enjoy the process.

2

The Magic of Beliefs, Values, Goals, and Persistence

You Can't Hit a Target You Don't Have, and You Can't Have a Target Until You Know Your Beliefs and Values

"Go confidently in the direction of your dreams. Live the life you've imagined."

—Henry David Thoreau

What's the difference between the person who continually tries to diet—or to get onto a permanent exercise program—and fails and the individual who steadfastly sticks with his/her program through good times and bad, the dieter who carries on despite demoralizing setbacks and temporary defeats and keeps up his efforts through thick and thin?

Is it physical or moral superiority? Is it finding the "right" diet? Is it unflagging support from family and close friends? Is it luck? Or is it an unremitting will to win?

While you could argue that all of these qualities are important, most people would agree that there is one trait that propels more dieters into the winners' circle than all others combined. That quality is *persistence.*

Persistence suggests a steadfast resolve that refuses to be compromised. It indicates a lack of self-pity and self-indulgence. And it implies above all else that unyielding "will to win," a refusal to surrender despite petty annoyances, major obstacles, even demoralizing setbacks. Whether you call it tenacity, stamina, guts, or determination, this uniquely human trait translates into that enviable quality of hanging on until victory has been achieved.

Our greatest victories are usually one step past our biggest failures.

The winners we see and admire in all walks of life have this kind of willpower. And the winners in the dieting game have it, too. They know how to learn from their failures rather than be defeated by them. They then use this new knowledge to reach even higher goals.

Conversely, lack of persistence is a leading cause of failure, particularly when it comes to making changes in diet or exercise. Sure, there are lots of people out there who want to boost their metabolism and get thin and fit, but not all of them want it *badly enough to persist in their efforts*. How about you? Are you willing to do what it takes, regardless of all obstacles?

Experience with men and women who have tried to kick their unhealthful habits has demonstrated that lack of persistence is a weakness that is common to the majority. They're ready to give up at the first hint of discomfort or pain. They're easily overcome by delays or setbacks. Only a precious few carry on, despite all opposition, until they achieve their goals.

Strangely enough, it is precisely at that point that most dieters could win the weight-loss battle. All they need is that little extra push to hang on for a short time longer. This thought was stated so nicely by the Greek historian Polybius:

> Some men give up their designs when they have almost reached the goal; while others, on the contrary, obtain a victory by exerting, at the last moment, more vigorous efforts than before.

Those who are persistent when it comes to behavioral changes earn their success at the very point where many other dieters end in failure. History is laced with examples where men and women have fallen short of their goals only because they failed to hang on.

How to Spot Weak Persistence

Take a look at your own history. You'll likely see that you've been victimized by lack of persistence in many of your previous dieting attempts. This has been the Achilles' heel of nearly all dieters at one time or another, and it tends to show up in a variety of disguises. Here are just a few:

- Willingness, perhaps even eagerness, to succumb to a temporary dieting slip
- Tendency to blame the diet regimen for your own inability to stick to it
- Fear of meeting head-on those situations which you know present great difficulty
- Inclination to compromise your dieting goals
- Failure to set clearly defined short- and long-term goals and hold yourself accountable for reaching each one of them
- Lack of an organized plan for achieving your dieting goals

Goal Setting Builds Persistence and the Desire to Win

A great example of a situation in life where persistence is essential is parenthood. After all, giving up is not an option when a parent is teaching a child to walk. Now let's make a similar commitment here: From now on, giving up is not an option when attempting to reach your health and fitness goals. From now on, you must rank being fit right up there with essential bodily functions such as breathing.

To reach this level of passion, you must have goals that are

- Perfectly clear and detailed
- Put in writing on some type of a goal chart so you can see where you have to be at every stage of the process
- Part of your everyday routine

> The most important aspect of reaching any goal is to work on its achievement, to the best of your ability, each and every day without fail.

Goal Setting Points the Way

Goals are the mental road maps that your mind uses to attain its desired ends, the conduits that funnel all of your physical and mental energies toward a single, important, *unified* purpose.

A wealth of professional research has shown that goal setting helps you focus on the tasks at hand and, as a result, improves your ability to stick to your behavior-change program. Writing in the *Canadian Journal of Behavioural Science*, researchers Pierre Baron and Robert G. Watters reported that dieters who set goals lose much more weight than those who do not. Their findings confirm scores of earlier studies on dieting, exercise, and behavior change, including those by Robert L. Litrownik of the University of Illinois and H. Jon Geis of the Institute for Rational Living in New York City. They all verify that the ability to stick to your program of change, no matter what its description, is aided considerably by proper goal setting.

How Goal Setting Builds Your Will to Succeed

Goal setting builds willpower by working in precisely the same way as "desire-building" exercises, in that both rely on the mind's ability to translate thoughts into concrete *things*, and ideas into successful *reality*.

Setting goals the *Maximize Your Metabolism* way keeps your new style of living at the forefront of your daily thinking. The result is that you're constantly reminded in a positive, yet forceful way that sticking to your diet and exercise regimen is your top priority, a daily routine to which you pledge unswerving allegiance.

Your goals become your mental companion as you steadily chip away at those unwanted pounds. They measure your successes, in effect complimenting you on your achievements, and direct your efforts away from past mistakes and false starts.

Goal setting is the best way to stay motivated. Goals provide focus for your workout program and clarify what you are trying to achieve. As you attain each goal, you are encouraged by your success, which in turn motivates you to stay the course.

Five Easy Steps to Setting Perfect Goals

There are five easy rules for setting effective goals. Anyone can do it. You need take only a half-hour or so, do a bit of soul-searching and pencil work, and—voilà!—you're all set.

Step One. Fix in your mind the *precise* goal you wish to reach, and make sure that it's something that's both measurable and specific. A vague goal, such as "I want to be fit," gives you nothing to shoot for. Decide when and what you are going to achieve, such as "I want to reduce my body fat by two percentage points by the 1st of September." Be sure to take whatever steps are needed to assess your progress. In this example, you need to know your current percentage of body fat (get it tested—it shouldn't cost more than $20 at any good health club) and then monitor it on a weekly basis thereafter.

But beware of a common mistake! Don't get caught in the trap of setting a goal for one thing when what you really want is something else. Many overweight people claim that they're dieting because they want to "get thin," even though their real goal is (or perhaps should be!) not simply to *get* thin but to *stay* thin. This is sort of like stating that your goal is to climb Mt. Everest when what you're actually aiming for is to build a six-room condo once you get to the top.

Since strategies for losing weight necessarily involve making changes in behavior, be as specific as possible about the extent to which you're willing to change your behavior. The last thing you want is to achieve your ideal weight only to complain later that the weight has come back. It would be much better to set a goal of reaching a certain weight and remaining there (within 2 to 4 pounds) for good.

Make sure that your goals are realistic and attainable. If you set your expectations too high, you will get frustrated and will be more likely to quit. On the other hand, your goals should not be too easy; they should be challenging. When you achieve a challenging goal, your pride and satisfaction will engender in you a greater degree of motivation to take the next step. Make your goals lofty enough to force you to venture beyond your comfort zone, but not so far from your current circumstances that they seem unrealistic or even impossible to you.

Put simply, set each of your goals at an appropriate level right at the outset. If you want to lose 15 pounds, say so. If you want to lose 40 pounds and remain at 110 for the rest of your life, admit it and be proud. If you want to lose 20 pounds and eat nutritionally better meals, let that be your decision. But above all, *be specific.* Tell your subconscious exactly what you want, and your subconscious will find a way to make it happen.

Once you have set a particular goal, don't share it with anyone for at least the first thirty days. That will give it enough time to sink deep into your subconscious mind and become part of your everyday life, a habit. After that, share it only with those people who you know will be encouraging to you and helpful in your pursuit.

Make sure your goal becomes such a burning desire that it drives you hard enough to fend off any negative feedback, from yourself or others, with virtually no effort on your part.

Step Two. Determine exactly *how* you are going to achieve your goal. This step of the goal-setting process calls for some planning on your part, since you've got to know how the *Maximize Your Metabolism* program will play out in your life.

Set short-term goals as steppingstones to your ultimate (long-term) goals. If your long-term goal is to be able to bench press 200 pounds within a year's time, set short-term (weekly or monthly) goals for the weight you will need to be able to bench press at each stage in order to achieve your long-term goal. In other words, develop a plan. It's a lot easier to limit yourself to thinking about accomplishing your goal just a little at a time, such as increasing your bench press by 2.5 or 5 pounds a week, than to have the specter of *the whole thing* (such as increasing your bench press by 50 pounds) hanging over your head.

One problem is that many would-be behavior-changers let other people think and plan for them. They *believe* they're actually doing their own thinking and planning, but they end up turning their problems over to others in the hope that someone else might solve them. Then they readily accept the opinions and decisions of others. Ralph Waldo Emerson noted this when he said, "Our chief want in life is somebody who will make us do what we can."

Step Three. Select a *timetable* for the attainment of your goal. Predicting the rate at which weight loss will occur, through caloric restriction and increased physical activity, will take some calculation and some imagination on your part.

Without a timetable to plot your course, it will be difficult to make firm connections between the fading past and the unseen future. To make this association more explicit, keep a logbook of your dieting progress. Although these dieting diaries are sometimes viewed as tedious, pencil-pushing exercises, they're quite valuable, not only for charting progress but also for reviving spirits that flag and re-energizing motivation that founders. Besides, it can be fun—perhaps even educational—to read them in later months or years.

Another way to track your progress is to get a piece of poster board and tack it lengthwise to a wall that only you will see. Draw a horizontal line across the center of the poster, and write your present weight at the far left side of the line and your goal weight at the far right side. Make tick marks on the line to indicate the weeks or months when you'll be "weighing in" or otherwise checking your progress. This will serve as a timeline, which you can use to visually track where you are now and where you should be at the end of each week or month of your journey.

Your weekly weigh-ins will keep you aware of your progress. Based upon the degree of your intermediate successes, you can either reward yourself or adopt whatever self-correcting behavior you need in order to achieve your goal on schedule.

Step Four. Decide what you'll do to prevent relapses in your program—and to meet them head-on if they occur. To accomplish this step, you'll need to deliberate and make contracts with yourself. Much of what you have done in your dieting past has been correct. Repeating your past dieting successes will bring you even closer to victory this time.

But what about those areas in which you've had problems? Do you find it hard to stick to a diet during holiday entertaining? Are you particularly vulnerable to dieting failure when you eat in a restaurant? Have you stumbled and fallen on your road to a fitter, leaner body as the result of a temporary personal problem (depression, anxiety, anger, etc.)?

Whatever the problem, you've got to *pre-plan* a solution for it, just in case it arises in your dieting life again. What will you do differently this time? Make a note of that action, and include it in your goal statement.

What I've found to be most effective is a process for enumerating all the foreseeable challenges that may arise and for deciding in advance how to handle them if they do. I originally developed this process for my clients, but I've used it in running my business as well. Here's how it works:

Go to any office-supply store and get a three-ring binder and a stack of plain, white, three-hole-punched paper. Using a separate sheet of paper for every challenge you think you may encounter on your way to reaching your goal, write out the challenge at the top. Below that, list all the undesirable consequences of failing to meet this challenge. Finally, write out the best, step-by-step approach you can think of to avoid being faced with this challenge in the first place (or to deal with it effectively if it does present itself and you happen to succumb to it).

Here's an example of what a challenge sheet might consist of.

Challenge: Eating out at a restaurant with friends

****

What bad can come of this:

1. I miss this week's goal
2. I lose self-confidence by giving in . . . and by thinking that just one bad meal won't hurt my progress
3. I reinforce my cravings and make reaching my goal that much more of an effort
4. ______________________________
5. ______________________________

****

How I can avoid this problem:

1. I can make sure that every food I order is on my diet, and I can tell the waiter not to use any butter or oil when preparing my food
2. I can pick a restaurant where I know I'll be able to order a special meal without any hassle
3. ______________________________
4. ______________________________

Step Five. The fifth and final step is to write a clear, concise success statement. Then, once you've written it, read it aloud to yourself three or more times each day, including once just after waking up in the morning and once right before going to bed at night. As you read your success statement, see, feel, and *believe* you have already reached your weight-loss goal, visualizing yourself from head to toe in top shape and full of energy, mentally and physically. Read the statement with feeling, and feel great when you say it.

Here's an example of what a goal statement might look like:

> I weigh 135 [or your goal weight], and I look and feel great. I love showing off my tight body. People congratulate me daily on my achievement. I reached my goal by following every step of the *Maximize your Metabolism* program.

Read this statement out loud to yourself at least three times a day. Memorize it. This is one of the most important psychological tools you can use to train your subconscious mind to help you reach your goals.

The Magic of Autosuggestion

What you are practicing in this part of our goal-setting chapter is the principle of autosuggestion, your direct link of communication with your subconscious. Here's how it works:

Your subconscious mind is always open and drinking in any and all stimuli from your surroundings. For example, your subconscious knows the exact color of the tree you pass after you make that right-hand turn just before pulling into the parking lot at your place of work. Your conscious mind may never have picked that up, but your subconscious mind picks up and stores everything. Just as easily as it picks up useless information, such as the color of that tree, it also stores everything you think about and everything you hear.

This is good news, for if your subconscious mind is open to everything you think and you can implant anything you want into it, then you can limit yourself to thinking positive thoughts and allow your subconscious mind to bring positive things into your life.

Now this book isn't meant to be an instructional guide to training your subconscious mind, but if you follow the basics outlined in the book you'll actually train your subconscious mind for success. And a trained subconscious mind is a powerful asset when it comes to gaining control of your metabolism and your health.

Each time you read your success statement, you are sending subliminal suggestions to your subconscious, suggestions which it *must* eventually heed. The more often you repeat your affirmation in a positive, emotional state, the faster it will sink into your subconscious. And remember: your subconscious mind reacts best to these suggestions when they are drenched in desire-supporting emotions and any other imagery from the five senses that you can provide.

One secret to really accelerating your progress is to take a large piece of poster board and make a collage of what your goal body looks like. One way to do this is to go through as many magazines as you can get your hands on and cut out pictures of bodies that look just as yours will look once you reach your goal. Paste them all on this poster board. Paste on pictures of entire bodies, as well as pictures of body parts such as a tight stomach or a great lower body. Paste on pictures of people who look great in street clothes or in a bathing suit. Paste on pictures of people who are enjoying life in their strong, healthy body. Then put this poster where you can see it on a daily basis, and keep adding to it. Above all, have fun with this exercise.

3

Your Burning Desire

The Starting Point of All Goal Attainment

"Whatever you persistently and passionately desire, is always fulfilled."

—Napoleon Bonaparte

Without a true, burning desire, nothing that is truly valuable and permanent can ever be accomplished—except, of course, by luck, and it doesn't pay to count on that. Once you have committed to achieving a goal and developed an intense desire, your brain begins to draw into your life the dominant thoughts that you hold in your mind. Success coaches have proved time and time again that your outer world is an exact picture of your inner world.

If you subconsciously focus on how fat you are, your mind will present opportunities for becoming even fatter. But if you have a burning desire to become more lean and energized, you will develop a stronger self-image—and your outer world (your body) will be affected accordingly. What is even more amazing is that the stronger your desire, the faster the results will become a reality!

Remember, wishing alone will never bring results in great numbers. Appropriate action must accompany those wishes. The first step is to develop a true, burning desire—so burning that it becomes an obsession. Next, you need to create a detailed plan of action for reaching your goals (or have a professional create a plan for you). Finally, you have to back up that plan with a level of persistence that refuses to admit of failure.

The information and exercises contained in this book are intended to serve as a set of blueprints to help guide you through the process of attaining a heightened metabolism, better health, and a more attractive appearance. Thus, you should use the book as your plan of action for reaching your goals.

Before we go any further, I'd like to share with you an exercise that helped me reach more goals in one thirty-day period than I had been able to reach during the entire year leading up to that time. I met a man who felt so strongly about this exercise that he instilled it in me. I have to confess that when he first described it to me, I thought it was going to be a waste of time. After completing it, however, I had a better understanding of myself and my desires, and I had my top four goals laid out in front of me. By the way, the goals that I developed in that process were far different from the goals I had thought were important to me prior to going through it.

The exercise is called Crystallizing Your Focus, because after you've completed it you'll have a crystal-clear focus of what your goals are and then we can proceed. Whatever you do, don't skip over this exercise! I assure you, its relevance will become clear as we continue.

Exercise #1. Make a list of 101 wishes for your body: things you'd like to change a little, things you'd like to change a lot, small alterations in your appearance, the way you walk, your strength level, your endurance level, your health (be specific), your energy level, your ability to handle stress, etc.

Take as much time as you need to complete this exercise, but try to do it in as short a time as possible. I've had some clients who have finished it in an hour, and I've had others who had to put in three days of consistent hard work to get through it. Do yourself a favor, and start when you have at least an hour of silent, uninterrupted time. If that means getting up an hour earlier than everyone else in the house in order to find the necessary peace and quiet, then that's what you should do.

Once you've completed the first part of the exercise, move on to the second part, which is far easier: "time prioritizing" your list. Next to each item, write a number that represents the amount of time (in years) you're giving yourself to complete each one. For example, if one of your wishes is to shed 25 pounds and you know you can do that in a few months, you'll write a "1" next to that one, because you know you can reach that goal in the first year.

Use the numbers 1, 3, 5, and 10 (for 1, 3, 5, and 10 years, respectively) to time prioritize the wishes on your list.

Okay, put the book down, right now,
and don't come back to it
until you've completed your time prioritization.

Great! Now you're ready to prioritize the items within each "time category" on your list. Just as in sports or other contests, you can make a basic tournament board to help in this process.

First, list all of your 1-year goals on one page, all of your 3-year goals on another page, and so on, until you have four pages (one page for each of the four chronological groupings). Next, take your list of 1-year goals and complete the tournament board: Take your first two goals, draw a box around them, decide which of the two is more important to you, and then write the more important one just outside and to the right of the box. Then compare that "winning goal" (the one you wrote outside the box) to the third goal on that sheet: put them both into a new box and choose the more important of *those two* goals, writing the more important goal just outside and to the right of *that* box. Continue this process until you have only one "winning" goal on that page. Then go through the same process and prioritize your 3-year goals, your 5-year goals, and your 10-year goals.

Stop right now and do the exercise.

Congratulations! You've now identified your top four goals for your body and your health. I'll bet you're a bit surprised by the results. If nothing else, you should be much clearer as to what you need to focus on for the remainder of this book.

Exercise #2. Now make a list of all of the things about your life that will improve once you've achieved your highest-priority 1-year goal. Things such as the new doors that will open up for you, the increased energy you'll have, the richer friendships you may have, the more confidence you'll feel, etc. Make sure to have at least twenty-five items on your list.

Now do the same for your highest-priority 3-year goal, your highest-priority five-year goal, and your highest-priority ten-year goal. Remember: list at least twenty-five benefits for each goal!

Now as you work your way through the rest of this book, I want you to focus all your efforts on your highest-priority 1-year goal.

4

Unleash Your Metabolism

Proper Elimination Begins with a Thorough Cleansing

One of the biggest difficulties that crop up in renovating the metabolic system is to undo the years of damage that's been done by eating the wrong foods, or by eating the right foods in the wrong amounts. It's bad enough that we've eaten all sorts of junk food, but far more problematic is that we've allowed way too much of it to accumulate in our digestive system, particularly in the colon.

Throughout the years, our bodies have digested and assimilated hundreds of thousands of pounds of food. That's truly amazing, isn't it? Even more amazing—and of much greater importance—is that unless we have consumed the correct foods, our bodies probably have not digested everything completely, at least not yet!

At different stages of our lives, our bodies react in different ways to the food we eat. When we began life, our systems were, for the most part, clean and efficient, and in our early years our parents probably fed us foods that were somewhat wholesome and promoted good health. As we entered our teens, however, our hormones kicked in, our digestive system changed, and the foods we chose to eat also changed—probably for the worse! As we got to the end of our teenage years and reached early adulthood, our enzyme production changed. Now doesn't it make sense that our eating habits should also have changed—*for the better*—to keep up with each of these various stages and changes that our body went through? Have yours? If you're like most people, the answer is a resounding no!

The trouble is, our enzymatic systems changed but our eating patterns did not. The fast foods that our teenage metabolisms devoured are now clogging up our slower, adult metabolisms.

Keeping Pace

Each time our body goes through a change, no matter how big or small, the consistency and the concentration of the enzymes in our system also change. Changes in our external environment bring about changes in our internal world. A dramatic but easy-to-understand example of this process is as follows:

Suppose you took two children, born at about the same time and in the same area, and both of healthy parents. Suppose, further, that you relegated one of them to life in a poor section of a third-world country while the other was brought up in the lap of luxury in a clean, healthful environment. Now I'd be willing to bet that if you took the well-off child to that third-world country to meet the impoverished one ten years later, the well-off child would become sick. Why would this happen? Well, the answer is simple: the child who was brought up in the healthful environment has never been subjected to the germs that he/she would have encountered in the impoverished country, while the less fortunate child has built up an immune system that allows him/her to literally digest the germs as they enter his/her body.

I use this drastic example to illustrate how changes in your environment can cause everything about your inner systems to undergo at least slight modification. This happens because the human body attempts to acclimate to its surroundings in order to survive. The same is true, though to a far lesser extent, in regard to changes in your age, your activity level, your sleep patterns, etc. Each one of these elements, if changed, would cause a slight modification in the production of enzymes in your system.

The Poisonous Result

When the human body is given the wrong foods on a regular basis, certain undesirable "matter" tends to build up on the walls of the colon. If this matter is allowed to remain, it ferments, and the fermentation may cause odors to emanate from either the skin (such as the skin of the feet) or the mouth. In addition to the fermentation, this buildup of matter is the main cause of blockage in the bowels, which is even more serious. In the worst case, blockages can cause illness and, eventually, death.

According to William T. Tiller, M.D., president of the International Association for Colon Hydrotherapy, waste material accumulates in the colon, and then it breaks down and becomes toxic. Waste particles are "toxic," in the sense that they are recognized by the body's immune system as allergens, so an inflammatory allergic reaction occurs, often resulting in one or another of a variety of disorders.

To avoid having this happen to you, the *Maximize Your Metabolism* program has been designed to gently remove these accumulated toxic wastes from your system.

As mentioned earlier, the longer this material is allowed to remain, the greater the buildup in the colon. This poisonous matter forms layers that are virtually "glued" to the walls of your digestive tract. The longer the layers are allowed to remain there, the more clogged the system becomes. In addition, this coating of dead material may start making its way up your colon, where it can cause even greater problems.

Constipation Provides an Important Clue

Fortunately, Mother Nature has a formidable warning system that sends out signals of imminent danger. As you might guess, that warning often comes in the form of constipation.

We've all experienced constipation at one time or another: abnormally delayed or infrequent bowel movements, or difficulty in eliminating dry, hardened feces from our system.

Although constipation is not a good thing, being constipated does not necessarily mean that we're in danger of toxic poisoning. But there are many people who are constantly constipated or are plagued with frequent bouts of this condition. Those folks should pay particular attention to this chapter.

The Cleanse

The answer to this problem is simply to "clean house"—our digestive house, that is. Cleansing the entire digestive tract once a week to re-energize the digestive system is recommended for everyone.

This process will scrape away at the built-up matter and eventually flush all of it away, allowing the system to function as efficiently as that of a newborn. The benefits that you can expect from this are abundant, including better sleep patterns; sharper concentration and focus; much less stress; stronger muscle contractions; better absorption of nutrients into your muscles, organs, and bones; and much more energy.

The most important aspect of this cleansing process is that it restores that born-again purity to your digestive system, thereby enabling it to maximize the metabolism-building features that will be introduced in the next stage of the *Maximize Your Metabolism* program.

The 24-Hour Cleanse

It's a good idea to begin each cleanse during the morning hours, with your first meal. The process itself couldn't be easier: simply mix the juice of one lemon into a glass of plain, fresh (preferably distilled) water, and then drink this mixture, being sure to wait at least ten to thirty minutes before you consume anything else. Think of the solution of lemon juice and water as a liquid Brillo pad, cleaning everything it touches on its way down. Though the overall cleansing process outlined in this chapter is to be done only once a week, taking this morning drink of lemon water is something you can do every day of your life for a mild daily cleanse of your digestive system.

Once you have drunk the lemon water and waited the requisite ten to thirty minutes, you may consume any fruit or vegetable you like, just as long as you juice it—but be sure to juice it yourself. (Bottled or canned juices are not allowed, since the processing removes many of the valuable vitamins and minerals.)

You may also prepare a vegetable soup by boiling pure water (no salt!) and adding fresh, raw vegetables.

Speaking of which, you should strive to buy the freshest, organic fruits and vegetables you can find. Organic fruits and vegetables have notably more vitamins and minerals, plus you get the added benefit of consuming food that has not been chemically treated in any way.

Drink Plenty of Water

In addition to the freshly juiced vegetables and fruits, and possibly a soup, you'll be consuming a fair amount of water on the day of your cleanse. Calculate your required water intake as follows: drink at least one cup of water for every 14 pounds of body weight. If you weigh 150 pounds, for example, you are to consume about ten or eleven cups of water. (The day after you complete the cleansing process, you may resume your normal daily consumption of water, which ought to be about one cup for every 20 pounds of body weight.)

Incidentally, when I refer to water, I mean *pure* water, not coffee, tea, flavored seltzer, iced tea, etc. In addition, no salt or salt products are allowed in the water you consume for your cleanse. As stated earlier, distilled water would be best, as it contains no harmful chemicals or metals. Although distilled water literally contains almost none of the natural minerals found in well water, it is still a far better choice when it comes to cleaning out your system.

What Else Do You Get to Eat?

Just one additional thing: during the cleansing period, you may consume as many fresh, raw, organic vegetables as you wish, and one serving of fresh, raw, organic fruit (but just one kind of fruit, no combinations!). Remember, the cleanse phase of this program is designed to give your digestive system a long-needed rest and purify it for the next stage of the program.

Keep in mind that many, if not most, of the people who undergo this cleansing process have overburdened their digestive systems for years. The all-American custom has been to eat whatever and whenever we want. It's not uncommon for people to start the day by eating a "hearty" breakfast of, say, bacon, eggs, toast, and coffee—and sending their digestive systems through a living hell as a result. Another common practice, which is just as bad, consists of skipping breakfast entirely—indeed, people who do this are depriving their metabolism of the fuel it needs to get fired up in the morning. The point here is that most people either start the day off by consuming the wrong foods or by depriving their bodies of food altogether.

Among other imprudent habits are big lunches full of all the wrong foods, snacking all afternoon long, a big dinner, and a full evening of nighttime "grazing" that often lasts right up until the time that the late-evening news comes on. People who engage in these sorts of bad habits cause their digestive systems to work overtime, getting virtually no rest at all during the "night shift" yet needing to be up and ready to go for around round of eating (most likely poor eating) the next day.

As you can imagine, the digestive systems of most folks want and need to be cleansed and recharged.

On the day of the cleanse, you can enjoy as many meals as you wish, as long as they consist of the following kinds of food: fresh vegetables or fruits and their juices; fresh vegetable soup; and fresh, clean, pure water. Nothing else should pass your lips during this portion of the program, things like aspirin and vitamins included. The only exception would be any drugs or other substances recommended by your personal physician or nutritionist. If you must take prescription drugs on the day of the cleanse, you should consult your physician in regard to the advisability of going through the cleansing process.

Why the Concern?

When you "fast" in this fashion, even for as little as twenty-four hours, any drugs you take could have a more pronounced effect on your system, since there will be no solid food for them to bind to, and no food in your system to protect your stomach lining from pharmaceuticals that may be too harsh for it. Many drugs, in fact, carry warnings about NOT ingesting them on an empty stomach.

During the cleansing period, you may experience a slight headache or some muscle soreness or stiffness. This is a normal response of your body to the massive amount of dead matter accumulated in your bowels. The more hardened material there is, the greater your chances of experiencing one or more of these symptoms.

Should you experience any of these symptoms, the most likely cause is the loosening of this caked-on material and the process of preparing for it to be eliminated. Shortly before the actual elimination occurs, the hardened matter takes on a more concentrated form in its attempt to survive. This makes the dead matter harder to eliminate, but it also signals its eventual breakup and elimination. Once the top layer of this built-up matter is eliminated, the layers below are quick to follow.

How Long Does This Process Take?

The total time that it will take to fully clean and eliminate this buildup varies from one individual to another. Some people can clean out their entire system in one to three days. Others have so much colonic "sludge"—for lack of a better term—that it takes them longer. If you fall into the latter category, my suggestion is to go through this "clean-sweep" process for three days straight, then refrain from it for a week, and finally repeat the whole thing.

Continue this cycle of cleansing and resting until you feel totally cleansed internally (physically lighter, more mentally alert, and more vibrant).

A sure sign that your cleanse has worked is expulsion of an abnormally large amount of feces in a single bowel movement. Another sign is having one bowel movement for each meal consumed in a single day; for example, if you eat four times on a given day, then you should "poop" four times that day, usually within thirty to forty-five minutes after each meal.

Your cleanse can last anywhere from one to three days. You may want to take a little longer than this on your first try—it's really a matter of personal preference. I suggest going through this type of fast on a regular basis, ideally once a week for a period of twenty-four hours.

Regardless of the time it takes for your initial cleanse to produce the desired results, going through this cleansing process will become easier and easier in subsequent weeks and your system will become cleaner and healthier as times goes on.

You can benefit from a weekly or biweekly cleansing for the rest of your life. Not only is it very healthful, but it also provides a great source of live enzymes and an ideal combination of nutrients for your body and mind.

Any diet that you start without first properly cleansing your digestive system is destined to provide few, if any, of the many benefits that you deserve to reap from it.

The Next Step

Now that your system has been swept clean of its impurities, we can begin the process of actually increasing your metabolism, and it all starts by changing the way you eat.

5

Taking Control

Your Blueprints for Losing Fat

Everybody knows how to lose weight and stay thin. Do you recall seeing the same sentence earlier in the book? The reason why I've reiterated it here is that, for years, Americans have been obsessed with only one side of the crucial dieting equation: the number of calories they consume. In one diet program after another, proponents have tried—and failed—to prove that reducing the intake of calories is the one and only answer to weight loss. Surveys show that 140 million Americans (about half of the population) are on diets right now but that 60 percent of Americans are overweight! Even worse, past studies reveal that a full 95 percent of those who are dieting will fail to achieve permanent weight loss.

To date, more than a hundred different dieting strategies have been devised. Most of them have been disseminated in book form, and virtually all of them claim that reducing calories is the Holy Grail, whereas nothing could be further from the truth. Your metabolism is far more important. Here's why.

We humans expend energy (calories) in three ways: by increasing our **resting metabolic rate**, by engaging in **physical activity**, and through the process of **thermogenesis** (the burning of calories that occurs when we digest and metabolize our food).

Resting Metabolism

More than half of the calories we expend during the day are burned up by a process known as resting metabolism or basal metabolism, which consists of the burning of calories for the

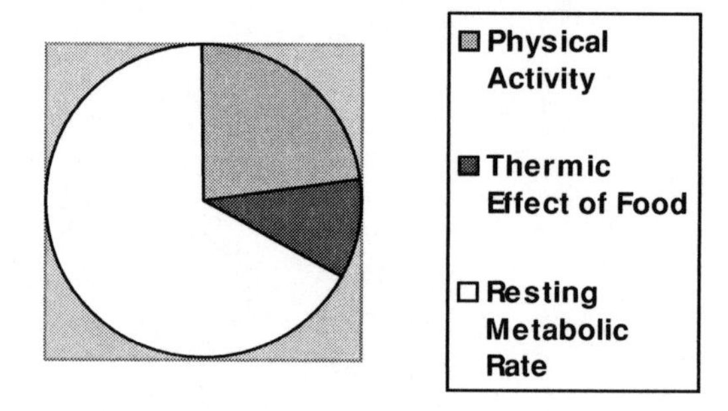

Categories of Energy Expenditure in Humans

purpose of producing energy to sustain life and maintain normal bodily functions such as respiration and circulation.

In an average male, resting metabolism is responsible for as much as 60 to 75 percent of the total calories burned. As we shall see in the chapters on exercise, however, resting metabolism is highly dependent on lean muscle mass and will form one of the key components that we're going to exploit in order to raise your metabolism over the long term.

Energy Expended during Physical Activity

The second component of metabolism is the number of calories burned through physical activity. Obviously, this is the element that most exercise professionals harp on relentlessly—and with good reason. This is one of the most significant variables in the metabolic equation.

The number of calories your burn during physical activity is dependent upon the frequency, intensity, and duration of exercise, and totals 10 to 30 percent of the total calories burned daily.

Most studies show that overweight men and women are less active, on average, than their physically trim counterparts. This is, of course, one of the major factors that cause people to become overweight in the first place—and to remain that way once they get there.

Thermic Effect of Food

The third element of metabolism is due to the thermic effect of food (TEF), which has to do with the energy we use up just by virtue of eating, digesting, and metabolizing food. As you might expect, this effect is most pronounced shortly after eating a meal. Indeed, the more calories we consume, the more calories we burn—in absolute numbers, at least.

In normal people, TEF raises the total energy expenditure of the body by more than 40% of the resting metabolic rate (RMR) within one hour after eating a 1500-calorie meal. That's about the size of a good Thanksgiving Day pig-out. The TEF typically peaks about an hour to an hour and a half after a meal, but it can remain elevated for up to six hours, depending on how calorically sinful your repast.

But don't get the wrong idea here: you cannot lose weight by eating greater quantities of food! The TEF is *never* enough to fully digest and work off all the calories consumed at a meal—in fact, it doesn't even come close.

Adaptive Energy Expenditure

There is one other element of metabolism that bears mentioning, and that is adaptive energy expenditure. This refers to the ability of the human body to *adapt* to stress or change. The effect of this component is not completely understood by scientists, but we do know that it varies from person to person and that it can play an important role in the energy-balance equation.

Because our body is highly adaptable, it actually responds to undesirable conditions by decreasing or increasing the amount of energy required for any given activity. It is for this reason that people in third-world countries are able to survive on a mere bowl of rice each day. Their bodies have responded to the lack of food by rigidly conserving energy and lowering their metabolic rate.

The Reality of Energy Balance

Being in a state of energy deficit, whether it comes about through decreased calorie consumption or increased calorie expenditure, will result in weight loss for *some* people. The standard formula states that to achieve a reduction of one pound of body weight, 3500 calories must be used up. The problem is that the more often a person experiences a severe energy deficit, the lesser the effect it has in the way of weight loss.

This adaptive effect is well documented through the experience of yo-yo dieters: the more they deprive themselves of food, the more likely it is that their bodies will squirrel away whatever nutrients they can muster up. Paradoxically, their self-deprivation makes it all the more difficult for them to lose weight.

Our body's survival mechanisms respond to intentionally inflicted calorie deficits just as they would during times of famine. That is, they become more efficient at using food by burning calories more slowly. What this means for dieters is that their metabolism slows down and they store the excess nutrients in the form of fat, saving it in case there's another deficit sometime in the future.

The best way to combat this natural tendency is to systematically increase your metabolism by every means possible, as we teach you to do in this book.

The human body is an incredible machine. It can withstand a great deal of abuse, and in time it will acclimate to almost anything that's inflicted upon it. We can train our muscles to grow (as when bodybuilders abuse their muscles by constantly increasing the amount of weight they lift, which forces the muscles to acclimate and grow in order to survive), and our brains to hold more information (the more we read and the more experiences we have, the stronger the neural pathways in our brains become and the more information our brains can process), and our lungs to hold more air.

Perhaps one of the most incredible examples of human adaptability is the power to train your metabolism to either speed up or slow down. And we're not talking about a process that takes months or years; we're talking about physiological changes that can be achieved in a matter of *days.* As healthy human beings, we can change the way our digestive system and our metabolism handle the food which enters our stomach.

Before a camel goes into the desert, it can store enough water to survive for weeks without a fresh supply. How does it do this? Well, I can assure you, the camel doesn't know how this happens, nor does it care. As long as it doesn't die of thirst, I'll bet it never even notices. A camel's system simply has a survival mechanism that triggers the sensation of thirst and increases the capacity of certain muscle cells to hold water. And the result? A rise in the amount of water the camel can drink and store.

Our Metabolic Systems Work the Same Way

If we deprive ourselves of water for some reason, our survival mechanism will cause certain parts of our bodies to store more water than usual. In fact, we will end up storing almost as much water as we take in. On top of that, the process of perspiration will slow down, thereby causing us to retain even more water. This not only makes us look "puffy," it also creates an atmosphere that is not conducive to achieving a heightened metabolism.

The solution is simple: In an earlier chapter you learned a simple formula that helped you determine how much water your body needs. Now all you have to do is supply it with at least that amount of water every day, causing the old, built-up water to be literally washed away.

The miracle of the human body doesn't stop there. If we can pull off this trick with our water-storage sites, then why not do a similar thing with the parts of the body where we store our carbohydrates, our proteins, and, yes, even our fats? The answer is that we *can*, and I'm sure you'll just love the way it's done: to train your system to shed fat, you simply need to trick it into believing that it will always be supplied with as much fat as it desires.

As great as it sounds, there is somewhat of a fallacy in this line of thinking. If the process of losing weight were really this easy, all you would have to do to reduce your fat content would be to ingest an abundance of fat, right? WRONG! Simply stated, what you have to do is see to it that your body gets the percentage of fat that it needs, not the percentage that your mind desires! Moreover, you have to follow a similar approach when it comes to your intake of carbohydrates and proteins. After all, too much of any nutrient will be converted to fat, a process that will simply prolong the entire fat-burning, metabolic-boosting process.

Remember, this is a training regimen. As with just about any kind of training, it may seem difficult, if not impossible, at first. Believe me, many of my clients have felt this way. However, what they quickly (and happily, I might add) discover is that once they take the plunge and get started on their new diet, they notice great results almost right away, and that's what keeps them motivated. Then, during their first week, they make a few minor modifications that help to tailor their diet, their exercise routine, and other aspects of their health and fitness so that they blend perfectly into their lifestyle.

To complete this training, we will need to teach our metabolism what to crave, what to use as fuel, and what to discard as waste. Our bodies now crave anything and everything that we enjoyed as kids. Unfortunately, since those days our metabolism has made a 180-degree turn-around in terms of what it needs to survive.

It is my estimate that nearly 90 percent of us have been eating meals that consist primarily of carbohydrates (breads, cereals, grains, pasta, fruits, and sugars) throughout our lifetime. This has trained our systems to crave and use carbohydrates as fuel. Then when we consume carbohydrates, our bodies assume that we are about to engage in strenuous activity. We are, in essence, like Pavlov's dog. Carbohydrates ring our bell, and our bodies respond just as they've been trained: they secrete a hormone known as insulin which will either (a) digest and use the newly acquired carbohydrates as energy, (b) properly store the excess in the liver or the muscles, or (c) deposit the excess in the form of fat. The normal action taken by the body when faced with strenuous exercise is to first use up carbohydrates from the stomach (the last meal eaten that day) and then go on to utilize carbohydrates from the muscles and the liver in turn. Only as a last resort will the body use up the carbohydrates that have been stored as fat.

The Road Back to Metabolic Health

To optimize our fat-burning furnace, we need to train our metabolism to go through a similar process whenever it sees fat, so that it will use that intake of fat as energy rather than immediately storing it in our cells. Since our metabolisms are accustomed to being positively reinforced for using carbohydrates as energy, this new process may be a rough transition, at least at the start. But you can rest assured that a successful transition will leave you with a body that uses up both the stored fat and the incoming fat as energy. And there are some rather nice side effects to all this: Your system will chip away at any cholesterol deposits you might have accumulated, and it will make better use of the vitamins you ingest. In addition, you will end up with a more abundant supply of vitamins A, D, E, and K, which are known to promote healthier hair and skin.

To accomplish this, you must gradually decrease your intake of carbohydrates, which will force your body to search for alternate sources of fuel. This decrease of carbohydrates must be accompanied by a gradual decrease of fat intake, which will force your body to use stored fat for energy, and a simultaneous increase in protein intake, to ensure that existing muscle is not burned as fuel. This process is not experimental; it has been demonstrated to work, and to melt off fat. Drastic forms of this approach, however, are unhealthful; therefore, I have provided an example diet for you later in this book.

Self-Monitoring Will Improve Your Success

When decreasing your intake of carbohydrates, your first step is to chronicle just what kind of carbohydrate-eating lifestyle you've developed. You can make the whole process easier by using one of those inexpensive journals, or even a small notebook. For the next seven days, keep a complete record of *everything* that enters your mouth (food, drink, snacks, gum, etc.). Then sit down in a quite place, where you're sure not to be disturbed for thirty minutes, and review what you've written.

You'll need to have four different colored markers for this project. Use one color for protein, and circle each and every item that is a major protein source (fish, meat, chicken, and anything else that used to be part of a live animal that has eyes, plus eggs). Use another colored marker to circle all of the sources of carbohydrates among the items listed in your journal, including any food that originated from plants (fruits, grains, vegetables, and beans) or is sweet tasting (for example, candy, cake, and non-diet soda). Use a third color for foods containing fats and fat products (butter, margarine, oil, mayonnaise, margarine, spray oil products, etc.).

Use the last colored marker to circle any items that contain a combination of nutrients from two (or all three) of the other categories. Examples of this would be fried foods (fried chicken contains both protein and fats) and baked goods (breads and pastries contain a combination of carbohydrates and fats).

Now look and see which colors dominate your list. My guess is that it will be your carbohydrate color and your combination color.

Next, over the course of the next thirty days, eliminate all of the fats (not just fats and fat products, but also fried foods). And don't object by claiming that your body needs some fats to survive. Unless you have some type of medical condition that requires you to consume a certain amount of fat (check with your physician if you think you do), you're going to be getting more than enough fat from the foods you eat, WITHOUT injecting ANY additional fat into your diet. In fact, your daily requirement of fat is a mere tablespoonful, yet the average American adult consumes six to eight tablespoonfuls of fat each day. Remember, our objective in this program is to force your system to metabolize your body's stored fat (for use in the form of energy) rather than to allow it to head directly for the food in your stomach every time it feels a need to supply you with energy.

Your body has had a valid reason for storing fat: you have been giving it so much fat, over so long a period of time, that you have convinced your body it will need this fuel for future use, and so it has stored it. Your body has only been doing its job.

In addition to cutting out all of the added fat from your diet, you must also lower your intake of carbohydrates over the next thirty days. During that time, you're going to eliminate all breads, pasta, cakes, sweets, sodas, and starchy foods (such as potatoes, beans, and avocados) from your diet.

In the meantime, you're going to increase your intake of leafy green vegetables (and other colorful vegetables), such as broccoli, peppers, asparagus, and cucumbers. To top this off, you're going to eat most of them in their clean, raw state, and you're going to try to get them from the organic section of your grocery store.

As if this weren't enough, you will also have to look at how all of your foods are prepared. Commit to not putting anything into your mouth unless it's baked, broiled, or steamed—or, in the case of vegetables, raw. If you go out to eat, as we all do from time to time, make sure that whatever food you order adheres to the above standards (it's really not that hard), and make sure that the person who prepares your food uses as little oil as possible in the baking or broiling process. (Eating food that's prepared without added oil is the best bet, but when eating out we must assume that the chef will add a bit of oil just for taste.)

The final aspect of your thirty-day changeover is the elimination of dairy products. The only food that's allowed in this category is egg whites. What this means is that for the next thirty day, you must refrain from consuming milk, cheese, and cream, as well as any and all products derived from those sources.

As an extra gift to your body, stop all alcohol and coffee intake. They're slowly poisoning your body and your mind by creating adverse chemical reactions.

6

Your New Metabolic Diet

Your Foundation for Metabolic Success

Now that we've given you a blueprint for losing fat, it's time to take a look at what a typical one-, two-, or three-month metabolism-maximizing diet looks like. The *Pyramid Program®* that follows was designed for any man or woman who wants to achieve a leaner, more energized, and healthier appearance.

You can use this program (which, as you will soon see, is actually a *three-diet* program) as a template, your template for dietary change. It was designed specifically for a woman who weighed 150 pounds. You can either use the diet *as is* or tailor the program modestly to suit your caloric requirements, whether slightly higher (for a rather overweight man, or for a woman who weighs more than 150) or lower (for a not-so-overweight man or a woman under 150 pounds).

As a general rule of thumb, you should increase or decrease your food intake by fifty calories for every five pounds by which your body weight differs from 150 pounds. If you take in fewer than the number of calories prescribed in this program, be sure that the majority of the calories you trim from your diet come from the carbohydrate category (that is, you should cut down on carbohydrates such as potatoes, rice, and breads). Conversely, whenever you increase your intake of calories, make up the difference either by selecting foods from the protein category or by eating vegetables that are especially good for your health (such as salads and raw, non-starchy vegetables).

The most important thing to remember is to eat according to the "Law of the Three ONLY's":

1. ONLY within the prescribed food groups

2. ONLY in the ratios specified
3. ONLY on the days scheduled

Getting Started

There are two phases to this program. The first phase will last from sixty to ninety days, depending on how quickly your body reacts to the combinations of foods you eat. Then you'll begin phase two, which is a "maintenance" step of the program. Phase two will supply you with the blueprints you'll need to either maintain your new physique or continue to lose weight. The maintenance phase is simply a time for you to begin adding back into your diet some of the foods you crave (within reason) and to balance the effects that those new foods may have on your body, so in phase two you should follow diet #2 (that is, the second phase-one diet) for a full two days each week.

Phase-One Objectives

The goal of phase one, which is the part of the program that consists of *three* separate diets, is to help strip fat and water from between your muscle and your skin while at the same time preparing your metabolism for phase two. Each of the diets in the first phase will bring you closer to your goal of total metabolic control in its own way. This phase has been designed to provide your body with the nutrients that are needed to burn any subcutaneous fat deposits, increase your energy level and metabolic rate, and improve your nutrient absorption.

Your New Food "Cycling" Program

In phase one of the *Maximize Your Metabolism* program, you must strictly adhere to diet #1 for two days, diet #2 for the following two or three days, and diet #3 for the final two or three days of a seven-day cycle, at which point you are to repeat the seven-day cycle.

It is this cycling of nutrients and calories that will enable your metabolism to attain its peak fat-burning level. While on this program, drink a minimum of twelve glasses of pure water each day. (I realize that this goes slightly against what I said earlier about consuming one glass for every 20 pounds of body weight, but for the time being, consuming the amount of water I'm suggesting here will help your body to shed fat faster.)

Here's what diet #1 looks like.

Phase One, Diet #1

Meal	Food
0	1 cup warm water w/ 2 tbsp. lemon juice added
1	2 servings of grits or cream of rice
	3 egg whites, large*
2	1 cup nonfat, sugar-free yogurt
	¼ cup Grape-Nuts *(optional)*
3	6 oz. turkey breast*
	1 mixed salad, large*
4	1 sweet potato, large*
	½ cup broccoli*
5	6 oz. chicken breast*
	1 mixed salad, large*
	½ cup brown rice*

*See the general guidelines that start on p. 55.

Again, the diets presented here are just examples. If you use these diets, you'll need to adhere to the following points, which you should apply to all three diets in this program:

- You should consume the warm water no later than thirty minutes after arising in the morning
- You should space the meals about two to three hours apart
- There should be at least one hour between the time you finish your last meal and the time you go to bed at night

Remember: each of the three diets is designed to be followed for more than one day during a seven-day cycle. Be sure that you consume *all* the foods listed for that diet on each of those days (and at the indicated meals). Don't omit foods from one day and add them to another day, and don't omit foods from one meal and add them to another meal.

Besides the solution of lemon juice and water (meal 0) that's to be taken every day, there are five meals (meals 1–5) to be eaten every day that you're on diet #1, and four meals (meals 1–4) to be eaten every day that you're on diet #2 or diet #3.

If you wish, a personalized diet can be created for your particular body—just visit us online for information about that.

Phase One, Diet #2

Diet #2 is intended to deplete your muscle stores of glycogen and water. Following this diet for two or three consecutive days will increase the rate at which your metabolic system burns fat. It will also reduce the capacity of your muscle cells to hold water, thereby causing them to release excess stored water.

Here's how you are to determine whether to follow this diet for two days or three days: If your weight loss is going a bit too slow, you should follow diet #2 for the full three days (and then follow diet #3 for only two days, in order to complete a full seven-day cycle for the three phase-one diets combined). If your weight loss is proceeding fast enough for you, then you should follow diet #2 for only two days (meaning that you would then follow diet #3 for the remaining three days of the cycle).

Phase One, Diet #2

Meal	Food	
0	1	cup warm water w/ 2 tbsp. lemon juice added
1	3–6	egg whites, large*
	2	rice cakes, plain*
2	6	oz. turkey breast*
	1	mixed salad, large*
3	3	slices fat-free American cheese
	5	fat-free crackers
4	3	oz. grilled meat*
	1	mixed salad, large*

*See the general guidelines that start on p. 55.

Since this portion of the diet program is low in carbohydrates, you may experience "withdrawal symptoms." Many diets that are low in sugar produce this effect, but it's entirely normal and there's no need for concern. This program was specifically designed to rid your body of such harmful elements as sugar buildup, toxins, and excess fat deposits. During the first two weeks, feel free to consume a small piece of fruit if you begin to feel overly lethargic or slightly dizzy.

Phase One, Diet #3

Diet #3 is designed for the final two or three days of your seven-day cycle. This food regimen will provide your muscles and liver with an ample supply of new glycogen in the form of complex carbohydrates and glucose polymers. Introducing these nutrients into your system at this point will force your metabolism and energy level to rise.

Phase One, Diet #3

Meal	Food
0	1 cup warm water w/ 2 tbsp. lemon juice added
1	1 serving of grits or cream of rice
	5 egg whites, large*
	spinach *(optional)*, in quantity desired*
2	1 6-oz. can water-packed tuna, drained*
	¼ cup brown rice*
3	6 oz. turkey breast*
	1 mixed salad, large*
4	6 oz. fish*
	1 mixed salad, large*

*See the general guidelines given below.

A more detailed description of these diets is found in the final chapter of this book.

When preparing your meals, be sure to avoid using any butter, margarine, oil, mayonnaise, prepared sauces, or salt. Instead, substitute any herb or herbal product you wish (just no salt or fat!). For the first two weeks only, you may also use fat-free salad dressing, fat-free butter, and fat-free mayonnaise, but there is a one-tbsp. limit per meal on these ingredients. Just in case you do opt to use these additional ingredients, you should be aware of the possibility that *they will slow your progress*. The only reason you're allowed to use them in the beginning is that they'll add a little taste to an otherwise bland diet.

General guidelines

No foods other than those listed on these pages should be consumed unless you first discuss any deviation from the *Maximize Your Metabolism* diet with your nutritionist or physician.

- If you are hungry or feel the need for additional food, you may increase your consumption of the protein sources (chicken, turkey, egg whites, tuna, and fish) at any of the meals for phase one during the first two weeks without slowing your weight loss.

- Either sliced or ground turkey (the 98% fat-free variety) may be substituted for chicken if you use it in the same quantity. Both chicken and turkey should be measured after cooking. Just in case you don't have a scale, 6 oz. of meat is about the same size as two decks of playing cards.
- While on this diet, you are permitted to consume any type of fish *other than* carp, herring, mackerel, mullet, salmon, sardines, squid, or tuna steak. These kinds of fish are simply higher in fat, and have been shown to slow the increase of metabolism in some people.
- For purposes of this diet, the term *grilled meat* refers to any very lean red or white meat (beef, pork, turkey, or chicken). As long as you're on this program, be sure that before you consume *any* type of meat, you remove all the skin and visible fat prior to cooking.
- For purposes of this diet, the term *mixed salad* refers to any combination of raw, non-starchy vegetables (one that's devoid of starchy vegetables such as potatoes, avocados, and beans).
- You may substitute a good "whey" protein powder for chicken/turkey or eggs, provided you make the substitution according to the following formula: two scoops of protein powder mixed in water is equivalent to either three egg whites or 3 oz. of chicken or turkey. Be sure not to make this substitution at more than one meal on any given day.
- Fish or sushi/sashimi may be substituted for tuna or chicken in this phase: 3 oz. of sushi is equivalent to 3 oz. of chicken or 1/2 of a 6-oz. can of tuna.
- Rice should always be measured *prior* to cooking.
- Vegetable quantities should be measured *after* cooking.
- A medium, plain baked potato may be substituted for 1/2 cup of rice. If you make this substitution, be sure to remove the skin from the potato prior to eating it.
- Candy that is both sugar free *and* sodium free may be eaten periodically throughout the day.

- For the first two weeks of the program, bagels, English muffins, and rice cakes can be eaten interchangeably, as long as you substitute one of them for another according to the following formula: two rice cakes is equivalent to either one medium bagel or one whole English muffin. You should be aware of the possibility that this substitution will slightly retard your weight loss.
- At some point during the first two weeks of this phase, you may experience a slight increase in intestinal gas. This is normal. It's caused by the elimination of previously built-up matter within your system, and the expulsion of this matter is an important step toward a fully functioning digestive system.
- You may experience an increase in urination and/or defecation during this phase of the program. This is due in part to the delicate cleansing effect that this particular combination of foods has on your digestive system, and in part to an increase in your metabolic rate.

7

Create an Energy Bang with Enzymes and Water

Immediately Boost Your Vitality by Increasing Your Digestive Efficiency

Do you want more energy without having to do any more work? If so, this will probably be one of your favorite chapters. After making just slight modifications in your diet, as outlined in the next few pages, your body and your mind could enjoy up to 30 percent more energy. What a tremendous boost to your health and to your life! Put into practice all the knowledge you gain in the rest of this book, and that percentage could go even higher!

What could you do with all that extra energy?

The human body uses more energy digesting food than it does in performing almost any other normal function. Thus, it might be tempting to think that if we stopped eating altogether, we would have endless energy (since none of our energy would be used up in carrying out the process of digestion). Unfortunately, that's not quite how it works. Our body is a very complex organism. In order for us to perform any action, we must first supply our body with enough energy (calories). Obviously, the way we do this is by eating and drinking. However, like a car, if the body is supplied with the wrong type of fuel, it will eventually stop performing, or at least stop performing efficiently.

This next paragraph is vitally important, so please read and reread it until you understand exactly why it has been included here.

In today's hectic society, we find ourselves spending less and less time thinking about the nutrients we put into our bodies. We do this so that we have more time to concentrate on work, family, and everything else. We then justify eating overcooked fast food, which dulls our focus and slows our physical and mental pace.

Hmm, what went wrong? Well, let me tell you: what went wrong is that we put way too little emphasis on the *types* of food we eat. If we simply spent more time in planning our food intake, the foods we eat could supply us with a much greater supply of energy, because our digestive system would require much less energy for the digestive process itself. It's no secret that digesting high-fat foods from fast-food restaurants requires much more energy than digesting foods that are more healthful. Choosing the correct foods, then, has a direct impact on our health and our energy level, because nutritious foods such as vegetables and low-fat proteins increase our metabolism and improve our immune and digestive systems!

This can easily be visualized in the following two sequences:

Poorly planned diet (fast food, for example)

→ More time and energy spent in digesting food

→ Less energy available to us, mentally and physically

→ Stress

Properly planned diet (low-fat protein and fresh, raw vegetables)

→ Fast, thorough digestion

→ Massive energy reserves

There are two nutrients that outperform all others when it comes to squeezing the most out of every calorie that we consume: *enzymes* and *water*. Enzymes have been called the spark plugs of life. They are responsible for digesting everything that goes into our mouth. Without enzymes, not only would our foods literally stagnate in our stomach, but our hormones and glands would be unable to function.

There are four major enzymes:

- Amylase, needed to break down starches
- Lipase, needed to break down fats
- Protease, needed to break down protein
- Cellulase, needed to break down cellulose

We need to have proper amounts of each of these four major enzymes—along with thousands of others, both known and unknown—in our system on a regular basis. When food, drinks, or other substances are introduced into the human body without the proper enzymes, those substances cannot be fully digested. Although the human body makes some of its own digestive substances, some foods cannot be fully processed without the help of outside enzymes that were "designed" to digest those particular nutrients.

Our Need for Enzymes

When a person eats red meat, the majority of enzymes necessary to digest that meat are not present in the meat itself. And for all we know, things may have been different in this respect a thousand years ago, before the introduction of steroids and other drugs that we routinely inject into our livestock nowadays.

Perhaps there were enzymes present in the meat back in the days when cattle were "free range" and were allowed to graze on the best of grasses, grasses that had not been fertilized with chemicals. Or when cattle were allowed to run free and to get enough exercise in the wild so as to remain strong, healthy, and free of the diseases that we find on the cattle farms of today.

In times gone by, the meat may have been full of the natural enzymes that are necessary for the human body to digest it in its entirety. But this is not the case today. The meat we eat is dependent on the intake of "outside" enzymes at the same meal for its digestion. If these other enzymes are not present, we are left with partially digested food in our digestive tract. Now the problem with partially digested food is that it becomes stale and stagnant, even to the point of developing gases and attracting toxins—and, eventually, even worms. (Yes, the human body can, and often does, provide a comfy home for various types of worms.)

The process that takes place in our digestive system is similar to what occurs when a deer has been hit by a car and is killed. After several hours, the flesh of the deer begins to turn rancid, which is similar to what happens when undigested meats are allowed to remain in the human digestive tract.

Why do I use such an unappealing example? The reason, very simply, is that I want you to get the point, and the point is that we need to digest our food as soon as possible after consuming it.

Retracing Our Steps

How do we do this? How do we stop this process of rotting and decay in our digestive system without taking red meat out of our diet? Simply by consuming the correct enzymes in the *same meal* as the meat! As stated above, protease is the enzyme that is primarily responsible for the digestion of protein, but we also need a sufficient amount of lipase in our system, since red meat contains a large amount of fat.

Is the mere presence of those two enzymes enough to ensure complete digestion? Absolutely not! Full digestion requires that those enzymes be combined properly, in a live state (such as found in raw vegetables), and mixed with other enzymes that facilitate their work. To get enzymes like this into your body, you must consume them in as *fresh* a state as possible.

One example of a food that has high levels of enzymes in its live state is raw vegetables. (And raw organic vegetables have a far higher level of enzymes than other raw vegetables.) Nevertheless, eating a few raw vegetables with a meal does not ensure full digestion.

Our bodies need to be healthy and "regular," as opposed to "constipated" (this was covered in great detail in chapter 4), before we eat meat. What this means is that you should *regularly* eat foods that contain high levels of live enzymes. As a matter of fact, a person who eats foods that contain high levels of live enzymes and omits all other foods from their diet (except for perhaps a small serving of protein several times each day) will be very healthy and quite regular.

Enzymes are found in all living things. However, they tend to get destroyed because of the chemicals we use to clean our food and the high temperatures at which we cook it. The foods that tend to contain plenty of live enzymes are fruits and vegetables, as long as they are eaten raw (not processed, canned, cooked, etc. before being consumed). Examples of foods that contain little in the way of live enzymes are meats, breads, pasta, processed or canned foods, etc. Virtually any process (including cooking) that we use to make food last longer or give it a longer shelf life is bound to destroy most of its live enzymes.

By now, it should be clear to you that without ingesting each of these enzymes in their correct proportions, we would fail to function. It is important to keep in mind that everything that our bodies ingest, no matter how large or small, must be either assimilated or eliminated, and both of those processes are controlled directly through our enzymatic systems.

The Magic of Water

Enzymes are not the only dietary component that we need as an aid in the digestion of the food we eat. We must also consume an abundance of plain, fresh WATER.

We all know how great a glass of ice-cold water feels and tastes on a hot day. But do you realize how absolutely important plain, clean water is to your health? Water is a rather simple organic compound, composed of two parts hydrogen and one part oxygen. It is tasteless, odorless, and clear, yet no living organism can survive for more than seventy-two hours without a constant supply of this largely overlooked miracle of nature.

The main constituent of the human body is water, to the tune of 70% by weight. Through stress or starvation, the body can become depleted by up to half of its carbohydrate, fat, and protein stores before death or disease sets in, but if only 20% of the body's store of water is depleted, delirium and death are likely to occur.

Your personal requirements for water will vary with your weight, physical activity, and age. The importance of the need to consume a certain amount of water was stated earlier, but it warrants repetition here. Under normal environmental conditions, the body of a physically active adult requires approximately one cup of water for every 14 to 20 pounds of body weight. This adds up to about eight to ten glasses of water per day for an average-sized female, and ten to twelve glasses for an average-sized male. To put it more precisely, the proper level of water in the body is attained when the input of water matches the output of bodily fluids. The main avenue for water loss is through the urinary tract, but the body also excretes water in the feces, in exhaled air, and through perspiration.

As stated earlier, water makes up over 70% of body weight in humans and is stored in various areas within the body. We will focus on two types of water storage in humans: intercellular and intravascular. Water that is stored intercellularly (literally, "between the cells") is responsible for the health of the cells that it encompasses. Unfortunately, it is also the main component of subcutaneous water deposits, which are deposits of water under the skin. This is the water that accumulates between a person's muscle and skin and causes the bloated appearance we all dread.

Water that is stored intravascularly (literally, "within the vessels") is the water that helps regulate blood pressure. When the body is deprived of water for an extended period of time, it compensates for this deficiency by moving water from one storage site to another, thus maintaining an equal balance of water everywhere.

The problem with this is that when water is transported from intravascular storage sites for use in other areas of the body, it causes the blood pressure to rise accordingly. Therefore, people who engage in strenuous activity such as sports without replacing the water lost through perspiration are taxing their bodies in more ways than they might realize.

In addition to creating an unhealthful condition in the body, a lack of water places the entire system in a survival mode, forcing it to retain any water that is consumed from that point on.

This is one of the reasons why nutritionists claim that people who have a greater-than-average tendency to retain water should gradually consume still more water—even to the point of throwing their body's defense mechanism out of commission—so that their system will begin to excrete the optimum amount of fluid. This takes the pressure off of the body and allows it to freely excrete both the old (stored or retained) water as well as the new water on a regular basis.

Whenever this balance is upset, the cells are forced to function with the old, more polluted water within them. As an analogy, think of your cells as inhabiting a lake. Now where would you rather live? In a lake that's stagnant and filled with algae, or in a lake that's constantly being "spring fed" with a clean supply of water? The answer is obvious.

Pure water should, by far, be everyone's natural choice of coolant and thirst quencher. Sodas and sports drinks that contain sugar (sucrose, fructose, glucose) and sodium actually increase the body's need for pure water. In a country such as the U.S., which is blessed with some of the cleanest drinking water in the world, it's hard to believe that most Americans consume far more carbonated, sugar-filled drinks than plain water.

The Enzyme–Water Link

Truly, the most healthful source of water available to us lies not only within our great water reservoirs but also within the foods those reservoirs allow us to grow. The most natural and most nutrient-rich state of both enzymes and water is their live state. Although that statement may sound a bit unorthodox or even gross, think of it this way:

A vegetable has a massive supply of both enzymes and water. Even better than that, those enzymes and water are combined in their most natural and most useful state. When we humans were created, we were given certain vegetation and animals to enable us to satisfy our hunger. Whatever your religious background, you must believe that those things were not given to us in cooked or chemically disinfected form.

Humans were designed to function at their peak level of efficiency, but that can come about only when the nutrients they consume are ingested in the proper proportion. Nature takes care of that for us by combining life-giving nutrients inside those pretty packages that we call vegetables, fruits, grains, fish, and meat.

Each of these foods just naturally contains the proper amount of enzymes needed to digest that particular type of food. The problems arise when we cook that food. Now don't get me wrong! I am certainly not advocating the consumption of raw meat. In fact, what I'm suggesting is more like the exact opposite of that.

What is so wonderful about this whole business of enzymes is that there is a major exception to the rule that each source of food contains virtually the exact amount of enzymes we need in order to digest it. The exception to that rule is the vegetables, which were endowed with a more-than-abundant supply of both water and enzymes. As a matter of fact, vegetables were given so much in the way of nutrients that if we were to consume them only in their *raw* state, we could get away with digesting quite a bit of the other four categories of foods in a *cooked* state. Thus, combining fresh, raw vegetables with all other foods is essential to the metabolism-boosting process.

8

Metabolic Superchargers That Work

Dietary Supplements and Metabolic Enhancers

No book about maximizing your metabolism would be complete without a few words on dietary supplements, since their use—and accompanying controversy—seem to be everywhere.

More than four out of every ten adults in the U.S. take vitamin and mineral supplements, or herbal and nonherbal concoctions that are thought to stimulate metabolism, curb appetite, or yield one of a myriad of other desirable outcomes.

As a nation, we spend more than $3 billion annually on supplements, making this category of products the third largest in terms of over-the-counter sales.

Hundreds of these products go straight to the heart of the dieting and weight-loss business, promising faster weight loss, higher metabolism, and a variety of other benefits ranging from enhanced sexual performance to fewer wrinkles.

What Are Dietary Supplements?

Dietary supplements are preparations—in many cases a pill, but frequently in liquid or powder form—that contain nutrients which are intended to supply the body with adequate, or more than adequate, supplies of what the body needs to function at a certain level.

Certain supplements can enhance your metabolism, improve your physical performance and health, alter your bodily make-up, and help you achieve a variety of other important goals. They're designed to help you achieve optimal nutrition, and to make up for the failure of most Americans to eat the foods that can provide appropriate daily levels of all the nutrients they need to thrive.

Metabolic Goals of Supplementation

In addition to improving overall health, supplements offer the student of good health an opportunity to focus on a number of goals specific to metabolic change, including increases in

- Muscle mass

  By increasing muscle mass, you increase your metabolic rate—by fifty calories per day per pound of muscle added!

- Muscle work capacity

  By increasing the aerobic and anaerobic capacity of your muscles, you heighten the amount of work your muscles can do, and you increase your fat-burning capacity accordingly.

- Energy expenditure

  By increasing your energy use, you increase the number of calories you burn each day. The more energy expended, the greater the number of calories burned.

Should You Use Supplements?

I'm often asked about supplements, and my advice is invariably the same: This program is founded on the principle that good health and maximum metabolism can be accomplished by increasing your energy expenditure in a certain way while decreasing your intake of certain foods and increasing your intake of others. However, you can accelerate the process by systematically adhering to a program of healthful supplement use at the same time.

Ultimately, the advisability and effectiveness of using dietary supplements comes down to the question of whether simply maintaining a healthful, well-balanced diet can provide all the vitamins, minerals, fiber, enzymes, and other nutritive components that you need to maintain vigorous and viable good health. Unfortunately, for most people the answer to that question is NO.

In today's society, the soils in which our fruits and vegetables are grown tend to be overused and are rarely given enough time between crops to replenish their nutrient content. And soil that lacks nutrients tends to produce crops that also lack nutrients. Top that off with the fact that in order to have a good crop season after season, farmers add literally tons of pesticides to our "natural" foods to ensure that the insects won't devour it.

A healthful diet is an essential start! Without that ingredient, we have nothing to build upon. An active lifestyle is a good second step toward attaining great health and a strong metabolism. Among the other components laid out for you in this book, you must also add a good source of nutrients to your daily regimen.

There are so many supplements on the market that I can't go into great detail about any one product, but I will say that in all my years of working with people, I've found only one type of supplement that truly encompasses every aspect of what we need as humans to survive and thrive, and that is a 100% natural, plant-derived, powdered nutritional drink.

There are many products out there that fill the bill. If you cannot find one in your health-food store, just contact my office and we'll help you find a quality brand. When you set out to look for a product of this type, make sure that the one you choose is composed of nutrients derived from a combination of several different sources, such as spirulina, barley, chlorella, seaweed, and other plants and herbs. Also, make sure that your product of choice is made only from organic sources. Then consume one, two, or three servings of this natural concoction each and every day.

I have been recommending this type of supplement to my clients over the years, for four main reasons:

- It's all natural
- You get everything you need in one delicious glass rather than having to take a handful of pills
- It contains all the nutrients that scientists have discovered, and possibly some that they have yet to discover
- It's 100% bio-available, meaning that every nutrient that's in each scoop you consume is assimilated and used to build the health of every cell in your body (as opposed to man-made supplements that are created in a lab, then pasteurized and dehydrated, and finally melted into a pill)

    Many man-made supplements are created from sources that the human body cannot assimilate. In reality, only 20 to 50 percent of what's in many of those pills is actually usable by your body.

The need for a nutritional additive in our diet should be obvious: the *average* American diet tends to be nearly devoid of the optimally healthful foods that I've mentioned—and way too heavy on fast foods such as hamburgers, French fries, and soft drinks.

Americans abuse their bodies nutritionally, thereby compromising their ability to absorb even the small amount of nutrients still found in the foods they eat. It's been said that a large percentage of people live most of their lives in a malnourished state—and are therefore plagued by chronic low-grade health problems, including fatigue, headache, weight fluctuations, sleep disorders, digestive discomforts, and stress-related difficulties.

Not only are our diets to blame for poor health. We've also had a series of formidable obstacles along our road to better health: pollution, stress, irregular meals, toxins and additives in our foods, and a variety of external pressures that, together, can push our body's systems to the edge.

Now bear in mind that you cannot take a crummy diet, add supplements to it, and assume that all will be fine. Nonetheless, let's move on to the topic you've been waiting for: supplements that actually help to increase your metabolic rate (as opposed to those that merely *claim* to do so).

There are a multitude of supplements that can help. The problem is that some folks find it difficult to separate the good from the bad. After reading this chapter, you will be able to make smarter choices for your particular needs.

What Are We Talking About?

Whenever I launch into a discussion about supplements, I find it helpful to draw clear lines about the category of supplements I'm talking about. At this point, I'm not discussing dietary supplements that are intended to provide a certain daily vitamin level. The importance of that type of supplement was pointed out earlier in this chapter. Nor am I addressing the myriad of pharmaceuticals and other medical preparations that are prescribed by doctors for their patients who need them.

This chapter is about the few supplements that can and should be considered for use in your program, together with a short discussion of some that should be avoided.

Individual Results Vary

Not everyone who uses dietary supplements will enjoy results that are identical to those that some friend or family member has told them about, but that's to be expected. After all, we're all different. The outcome of supplement use will vary according to such things as genetic factors; your body's ability to digest, absorb, and utilize the particular supplements you ingest; your current state of health; and your past and current dietary habits.

The bottom line is that in using supplements, each of us is undertaking an experiment. Try some of the supplements that you think may be helpful to your program, and then evaluate your results over time, closely following the manufacturer's and your doctor's recommendations.

Let's start by taking a look at a few of the safe and possibly helpful supplements.

Chitosan

Chitosan is a naturally occurring substance derived from chitin, which is found in the exoskeleton of shellfish such as shrimp or crabs. While it's chemically similar to the plant fiber known as cellulose, studies indicate that chitosan may have an advantage over cellulose (namely, that it may bind to fat before that fat has a chance to become metabolized). Researchers have speculated that the way it works is to convert to a gel in the stomach and "trap" the fat, thereby preventing its absorption and subsequent storage. Both the chitosan and the fat are then excreted in the stool.

In addition to absorbing fat to promote weight loss, chitosan also inhibits the formation of bad cholesterol and boosts the formation of good cholesterol. Its promoters also say it can be helpful in the healing of ulcers and lesions.

Chromium

Chromium is an essential trace mineral best known for its role in the metabolism of glucose. Its chief use as a supplement is to enhance glucose digestion and the body's ability to burn fat.

The typical American diet—one that is dominated by processed foods—is not rich in chromium-containing foods, such as whole grains. In fact, such diets are not only low in chromium, they are actually chromium *robbing*, because consuming too many processed foods depletes the body's supply of chromium.

Chromium picolinate is a combination supplement that helps regulate your sugar levels and lowers your LDL (bad cholesterol) level. Studies have shown that chromium may eliminate fat while at the same time increasing lean muscle. This is why chromium picolinate is such a popular supplement among athletes and those who engage in strength-building exercises. Chromium also promotes the metabolism of glucose, and it helps people achieve some of the most important results they're looking for when they embark on a weight-loss diet: a lowering of body fat, an increase in lean-muscle tissue, and a diminished craving for sweets and sugar.

L-carnitine

L-carnitine is an amino acid and an essential cofactor in the production of energy from fats (lipids). Strength-builders can benefit from L-carnitine, since the substance's ability to utilize fat in the production of energy can prevent muscle-protein loss during heavy workouts.

L-carnitine occurs naturally in the body and can be found in meat or meat extracts. Supplementing your body's supply of L-carnitine may aid in weight loss and fat reduction and promote muscle development, thereby speeding up your metabolism. It also helps to prevent a variety of illnesses, such as liver and kidney disease or diabetes, and to relieve symptoms of several diseases, including neurological diseases associated with aging, immune-system dysfunction, and diabetes.

Citrimax

Citrimax contains hydroxycitric acid (HCA), which acts as an appetite suppressant. Studies show that Citrimax may even prevent carbohydrates from being converted to fat.

Citrimax has also been said to lower the production of both cholesterol and fatty acids as a result of its effects on metabolism, and to do so **without adversely affecting the central nervous system or causing undesirable side effects** such as anxiety or jitters.

Gymnema sylvestre

Gymnema sylvestre is an herb found in tropical India that reportedly lowers blood sugar and enhances the activity of anti-diabetic drugs. The herb is also said to block glucose from being absorbed by the intestines, so it enables sugar to pass through the body.

The apparent safety of gymnema sylvestre is based primarily on its long use in traditional Ayurvedic medicine, where no serious adverse effects have been reported. It has been used for thousands of years to suppress the effects of high sugar intake.

Bitter melon

The bitter-melon fruit is widely used as food, as well as medicine, in Asia. The bitter melon is an anti-diabetic, which has been shown to increase the number of beta cells in the pancreas, thereby improving the body's ability to produce insulin. It is one of the few agents that have the potential to bolster a flagging pancreas.

At least three different groups of constituents of bitter melon have been reported to have blood-sugar-lowering effects, which may be of benefit in controlling diabetes mellitus. These active constituents are believed to prevent absorption of sugar by the intestines.

Citrus aurantium

Citrus aurantium has been shown in some recent studies to help stimulate the body's ability to use up calories by generating heat (thermogenesis). Citrus aurantium helps the body to effectively utilize stored fat, elevates the metabolic rate, and helps suppress appetite.

Hydroxycitric acid (HCA)

HCA (also mentioned earlier, in the description of Citrimax) is a natural compound extracted from the rind of the fruit of the garcinia cambogia tree, which is native to India and is also known as brindle berry. HCA inhibits the enzyme responsible for turning carbohydrates into fat, and it increases the ability of the liver and muscles to store glycogen, which suppresses your craving for carbohydrates by tricking your brain into thinking that your body's carbohydrate stores are full. HCA has been found to be effective in reducing fat production. In numerous studies it has also been shown to inhibit the conversion of excess carbohydrates and sugar into fat, as well as to suppress appetite and reduce body weight.

Guggulipid

Gugglesterone (also known as guggulipid) is a nutrient that is essential to the proper metabolism of cholesterol. Several studies have shown that guggulipid can decrease triglycerides (fats) as well as LDL (bad cholesterol) levels while increasing HDL (good cholesterol) levels in human subjects. Apparently, the way it goes about regulating cholesterol is by causing an increase in thyroid hormone levels (both T4 and T3).

Studies have also shown gugglesterone to be a fat-reducing compound. Athletes often use this supplement, because it is said to reduce joint inflammation and to help decrease joint discomfort caused by exercising.

Gugglesterone also provides needed substrates for the production of neurotransmitters (epinephrine and norepinephrine) that are involved in bringing about weight loss and in regulating metabolic rate.

Phosphatidyl choline

Phosphatidyl choline is a naturally occurring molecule that is composed of choline, phosphoric acid, and hydrocarbons. It is one of several phosphorus-containing lipids that form the structural elements of all cell membranes in the body.

Besides promoting proper functioning of the nervous system, choline is needed to metabolize fats and to help the liver function normally. Without choline, fats get trapped in the liver and block metabolism. In animals, choline deficiency results in an impaired release of fats, resulting in obesity. For these reasons, choline has been classified by scientists as an essential nutrient for humans.

5-HTP

5-HTP is used by the human body to make serotonin, a neurotransmitter which is vital to brain function. Serotonin is a chemical that is significantly involved in mood stabilization and appetite control, so it can provide a sense of calmness and steadiness of mood. Serotonin also appears to play a significant role in sleep, pain control, intestinal peristalsis, and other body functions, and to reduce inflammation.

5-HTP is not present in significant amounts in a typical diet. Supplemental 5-HTP has been shown to be effective in decreasing the need for carbohydrates and fats and in promoting weight loss.

Supplements That Are Cause for Concern

While there are many dietary supplements that are extremely helpful in promoting metabolism and weight loss, there are also supplements and chemicals that you may do well to avoid. The list that follows contains nutrients and/or drugs that I do not suggest taking. If you follow the guidelines in this book, you will get the results you want without resorting to the use of potentially harmful substances such as the ones on this list.

Ephedrine

One such supplement that has drawn relentless medical disapproval is ephedrine. Many men and women seeking the benefits of fast and easy weight loss succumb to the advertising claims made about the use of ephedrine-based supplements as a diet and exercise "super booster." Ephedrine acts primarily as a thermogenic aid but is also marketed as an energy booster.

The folks who buy into this line of marketing often find that a horrific cocktail of medical problems awaits them, either now or in the future. Ephedrine-based fat burners do work for some dieters, but the benefits are often paid for in the form of a rising tide of illness. For example, it is not uncommon for a person using ephedrine to report mild to severe side effects, such as chest pain, dizziness, and insomnia.

What is ephedrine?

Ephedrine is harvested from a plant called ephedra. There are some forty different species of ephedra, and it grows in regions of Asia, Europe, North America, and South America. Chinese ephedra plants are known as ma huang, the name by which ephedrine itself is commonly known. Though ephedrine is the most popular weight-loss supplement in the U.S., its use is very controversial. It has been shown to help people lose weight by jacking up the metabolism, so that the body will burn more calories. To a lesser extent, it causes suppression of appetite.

How it works

You've heard of the fight-or-flight reaction, right? In case you haven't, it's your sympathetic nervous system's response to a stressful situation. Your system gears up to either go into battle or escape a situation immediately.

Physiologically, the heart rate and blood pressure increase to prepare the body for action. Ephedrine mimics the effects of epinephrine and norepinephrine, the two naturally occurring chemicals in the body that are primarily responsible for the fight-or-flight reaction. When you take ephedrine, what you're basically doing is stimulating your sympathetic nervous system, which has the following effects:

- **Increased heart rate** and an increase in the force with which the heart contracts
- **Increased blood pressure**, sometimes accompanied by thickening of the blood
- **Increased rate of thermogenesis**, the process of the production of heat which is generated by the systemic burning of calories
- **Increased flow** of blood to the brain
- **Slightly increased** basal metabolic rate

Ephedrine interacts with many other substances and can be potentially dangerous for users with a pre-existing medical condition (in many cases, a condition of which they are unaware).

Adverse reactions to ephedrine include increased blood pressure, arrhythmias (heart-rate irregularities), insomnia, anxiety or nervousness, tremors, headache, seizures, heart attack, and stroke. The FDA has received hundreds of reports of adverse reactions linked to ephedra, ranging from mild effects such as a racing pulse, sweating, or a tingling sensation to sometimes-deadly cases of heart attack and stroke.

Androstenedione

Androstenedione (chemically known as 4- or 5-androstene-3beta, 17beta-dione) is a steroid hormone that is the precursor to testosterone, the steroid hormone associated with masculinity.

When taken orally, this chemical slightly increases blood levels of testosterone. As with other steroid hormones, androstenedione slightly improves the body's ability to recover quickly from strenuous exercise, thus allowing an individual to train more intensely. Those who are in the business of selling this substance promise an increase in muscle size and strength—and, accordingly, higher metabolism. This theory, however, is still up for grabs.

A study reported in the *Journal of the American Medical Association* suggests that androstenedione does not, in fact, increase testosterone but unfortunately *does* increase LDL cholesterol (the bad cholesterol). LDL cholesterol is believed to increase the risk of heart disease and stroke. Although use of androstenedione is legal in the U.S., it has been banned by some sports federations, including the National Collegiate Athletic Association.

Guaraná

Guaraná is a tropical plant that bears small red fruit. The people of the Amazon region in Brazil use guaraná as a source of energy, by either chewing the seeds or drinking the powder dissolved in water.

In the U.S., guaraná powder can be found in health-food stores. It's often used to boost stamina and endurance, or to help a person stay wide awake and alert. Promoters also claim that guaraná can help alleviate intestinal problems such as diarrhea.

The problem with guaraná is that it is very high in caffeine, so extreme care should be taken to avoid overuse. Caffeine, of course, has been linked to a variety of medical problems, including central nervous system disorders, certain cancers, osteoporosis, and other ailments.

What Else Is Recommended

While the outlandish claims made about some supplements tend to cast a shadow on the supplement industry as a whole, an increasing number of experts, including many doctors, suggest that many people can benefit from dietary supplements, particularly if they are taken in conjunction with a nutritionally sound diet and exercise regimen. One thing that's important to keep in mind, however, is that both the amount of weight loss and the risk to health and safety will vary from one dietary supplement to another.

What I advise my clients to do is to eat the *foods*—rather than to just take supplements—that contain the essential vitamins, minerals, and enzymes that are needed for proper metabolism. This is not to say that proper vitamin supplementation is not beneficial, but you should first look to foods to fulfill your vitamin and mineral needs, and then supplement where necessary.

For example, all nutrients are vital for maximum metabolic energy, but optimal levels of all B-complex vitamins are *especially* important, since they're cofactors in all metabolic functions. The

B vitamins work in concert with various enzymes that break down carbohydrates, proteins, and fats, as spelled out here:

- **Vitamin B1** serves as a co-enzyme in the metabolism of carbohydrates
- **Vitamin B2** is a must for cellular respiration, as is vitamin B3 (also known as niacin)
- **Vitamin B5** helps to ensure that our adrenal glands function properly
- **Vitamin B6** is needed for the metabolism of carbohydrates, proteins, and fats
- **Vitamin B12** plays such an important role as an energy booster that a proper discussion of it would take up an entire chapter all by itself

  One of the important functions of vitamin B12 is to help prevent anemia, which can decrease the amount of oxygen delivered to the brain and other parts of the body; it is also critical to the synthesis of DNA.

Vitamins B1, B2, B3, and pantothenic acid are particularly important for anyone who undertakes the program of physical activity that I'm recommending in this book. Deficiencies in these nutrients often result in fatigue and a reduced aerobic capacity, which is caused by the inability of the body to metabolize the lactic-acid by-products of heavy exercise.

In addition, vitamin B12 has been found to be essential to proper metabolic activity. This vitamin also seems to help neutralize adverse reactions to the sulfite preservatives that are found in so many foods and beverages and are responsible for life-threatening asthmatic attacks in sensitized individuals.

Special Provisos for Those Who Use Supplements

If you decide to use dietary supplements—and I suggest that you consider doing so—a few additional words of caution could be helpful:

- Check with your doctor to be sure that safe for you to take the specific supplements you have in mind
- Use each supplement as directed
- Avoid taking supplements in "mega" doses (ten or more times the recommended Daily Value)

9

Lift More Now, Weigh Less Forever!

The Power of Anaerobic Training and Muscle Stimulation

Ask any American what comes to mind when he or she thinks of exercise, and most will reply with the name of some form of *aerobic* exercise, such as bicycling, swimming, or cross-country skiing. Ever since Dr. Kenneth Cooper's first book, *Aerobics*, was published in 1968, the benefits of aerobic exercise have been widely touted. In fact, the fitness boom of the 1970s and 1980s coincided with the rise in aerobic exercise, especially recreational running and jogging.

Aerobic exercise can bestow many benefits on those who engage in it, including increased lung capacity and improved heart function, both of which help supply oxygen to the working muscles and improve the health of your heart and cardiovascular system. But aerobic exercise does little to develop or maintain *muscular strength*. And while aerobic exercise is important to a top-flight metabolism, it takes a back seat to strength training when it comes to controlling the *way you go about* burning calories and losing weight as well as the *amount* of weight you lose.

The next few chapters were designed to give you a clear understanding of how certain types of exercise affect the functioning of your body and what you can do to gain control. You must learn both of these if you are to truly maximize your metabolism.

Strength Training Induces A Higher Metabolic Rate

The term *strength training* refers to developing muscle strength and endurance through resistance training. *Muscle strength* refers to a one-time maximum effort of force that one applies in an isolated movement of a single muscle group. Technically defined, *muscle endurance* is the ability of muscles to apply a sub-maximal force repeatedly or to be exercised over an extended period of time. Common exercises that build both muscular endurance and strength are push-ups, sit-ups, chin-ups, a variety of machine exercises, and lifting of free weights.

Strength training will prevent muscle tissue from declining as you get older. Contrary to popular myth, however, strength training will not make you bulky unless you set up a strenuous program that's geared to that particular purpose.

Keep in mind that the chief metabolic difference between aerobic exercise (exercise that uses oxygen *during* performance) and anaerobic strength-building exercises is that while aerobic exercise burns more body fat *during* the actual exercise session, anaerobic exercise continues to cause calories and body fat to burn for quite a while after the exercise session is over. For this reason, anaerobic exercise has a far more dramatic effect on your resting metabolic rate. You'll see why in a moment.

Scientists have only recently begun to recognize this benefit of anaerobic exercise. Training for muscular strength has long been popular among bodybuilders and professional athletes, but it is only now finding its way into the workouts of other Americans. The evidence is now clear that muscle-enhancing exercises offer health and fitness benefits that everyone needs.

Metabolic Benefits of Strength-Building Exercise

One of the principal benefits of strength training is that it builds the density of muscle—and the denser the muscle, the more calories that are burned up. Losing muscle but continuing to take in the same amount of food forces people to put on weight in the form of body fat.

Unfortunately, that's precisely what tends to happen to us humans over the course of our adult life. As we age, our metabolism decreases by about one-half of one percent per year. When we reach our thirties, we begin to lose muscle mass, so we'll just naturally gain weight unless we take measures to prevent it from happening. Considering that every pound of muscle burns up to fifty calories a day, it's easy to understand the contribution that muscle mass makes to losing weight quickly and effectively—and keeping it off in the long run.

The *Maximize Your Metabolism* program is intended to help you build a strong metabolism, decrease your body fat, and increase your muscle density, but not to increase your weight. Although muscle weighs more (per unit volume) than body fat, muscle takes up far less space. Thus, the end result of going through this program will be a much slimmer, tighter, more efficient, and healthier body.

Traditionally, it was thought that metabolic balance—and therefore weight maintenance—could be achieved through a simple balance of energy sources: Input had to be commensurate with output. If you consumed more calories than you burned, you would *gain* weight; if you burned more calories than you ate, you would *lose* weight. In order to maintain a given weight, the number of calories consumed had to equal the number of calories spent.

Although this was a sound theory, it failed to take into account the body's awesome ability to adapt. It is now widely recognized that adaptation is one of the important functions of our rather sophisticated metabolic system.

The Reality of Energy Balance

The creation of an energy deficit, either through decreased calorie consumption or increased calorie expenditure, will result in weight loss for most people. Unless this is done properly, however, weight loss will probably be achieved *only the first few times a person creates an energy deficit*—and even *then*, the weight loss isn't likely to be long lasting. For every 3500 calories of energy used up, there should be a reduction in body weight of one pound. The more often a person experiences a severe energy deficit, however, the less of an effect it has on weight loss.

This adaptive effect is well documented through the experience of the yo-yo dieting generation. The greater and/or more frequent the energy deficit, the more difficult it becomes to lose weight (and the easier it is to gain weight!).

Our body's survival mechanisms respond to drastic calorie deficits just as they would during times of famine. That is, they become more efficient at using food energy, by burning calories more slowly. What that means for the dieter is that when they consume greater quantities of food, their slower metabolism causes the excess nutrients to be stored as fat, which the body wants to save in case there's another deficit sometime in the future.

Let me repeat this very crucial point: The more instances in which you restrict your calorie intake for a prolonged period of time, the slower your metabolism becomes. The slower your metabolism becomes, the more calories your body will store as fat the next time you eat.

The best way to combat this natural tendency to conserve energy is to reset your metabolic rate with a comprehensive program of strength building and aerobic activity. Both types of exercise are vital to firing up your metabolism. What will help you make permanent weight loss a part of your life—and give you a greater sense of personal satisfaction as a result—is a *balanced* fitness program.

Strength Training to the Rescue

While it is common knowledge that aerobic exercise is crucial in helping the overweight shed unwanted pounds, a growing portion of the research in the field of health and fitness suggests that strength training plays an especially important role.

Wayne L. Wescott, Ph.D., a physician and author of several popular fitness books as well as a former YMCA fitness director, is one of the leading proponents of strength training. His research—the results of which are consistent with my own findings—shows that dieters who engage in both strength-training exercise and aerobic exercise lose significantly more weight than those who limit themselves to aerobic exercise alone. This greater weight loss in those who take up strength training stems from a combination of greater expenditure of calories and a heightened metabolism that burns fat throughout the day.

According to Wescott, these dramatic results can be traced to the metabolic differences between muscle and fat. "Muscle is very active tissue," says Dr. Wescott, "and requires more energy to maintain than fat."

The trouble is that as we grow older we lose valuable muscle mass. Physiologists estimate that every pound of muscle we lose reduces our RMR by up to fifty calories a day. That's bad, and we need to retake control by replacing that lost muscle mass via a regular strength-training program.

As we age, Dr. Wescott explains, our RMR naturally decreases by about one-half of one percent per year. Thus, if we continue to eat the same types of food that we did when we were younger—and in the same amounts that we did then—we'll automatically gain body fat, unless we take preventive measures. Indeed, we will not only add body fat but also lose vital muscle density and strength. As a result, our bone density will be lowered, the health of our internal organs (including our heart) will decline, and our mental clarity will suffer. As you can see, in touting only the weight-loss benefits of including both aerobic and anaerobic exercise in a daily fitness regimen, we're really just scratching the surface in terms of the good that can accrue.

When the overweight depend on diet alone to control weight, what often happens is that they lose muscle, not fat. In fact, up to 50 percent of weight loss that results from dieting alone can manifest itself in the form of loss of lean muscle. This poses an enormous problem: Lean muscle burns calories, even while the body is at rest, while fat *stores* calories. The more fat we store, the easier it can be to gain weight. Strength training turns this situation around by helping us to shed fat.

The Metabolic Good News

For every pound of fat that you replace with muscle, you'll *lose* half a pound of body weight. Replace ten pounds of fat with muscle, and you'll notice *enormous* changes in your fat-burning potential, as well as in your ability to eat greater amounts of food without gaining weight.

Best of all, strength training provides results *quickly*; it can help you add over a pound of muscle *each month* that you're in training. In just a few months, you can rebuild the muscle you may have lost over the years as a result of a sedentary lifestyle.

The upshot of all this is that people who try to control their weight through diet *alone* can still have the metabolism of a "fat" person, even if they have a temporarily thinner body. And when these people resume normal eating, they often find that the old weight returns—this time with "interest," in the form of added pounds, leaving them even heavier than at the start. This can ultimately lead to the yo-yo syndrome: ongoing fluctuations in body weight.

It is far more efficient to use *exercise* (rather than *diet*) as a metabolism-boosting and fat-burning strategy. We burn off calories both *during* and *after* exercise—even as we sleep, watch television, or read a book. Strength-building exercises fire up our caloric "furnace" and raise our resting metabolic rate. And that's not all!

What Happens When You Weight Train

Physiologically speaking, when you engage in strength-training exercises, your body causes your muscle tissue to break down. In a sense, you actually *injure* your muscle tissue. Then when you rest the affected muscles and supply them with the proper nutrients, they automatically seek to protect themselves from further injury by becoming stronger and more responsive.

This may sound like a harsh—perhaps even a masochistic—way to set about losing weight, but it's totally natural and actually very healthful. Your body adapts to stress by repairing its muscle tissue and stimulating new muscle-tissue growth to overcome the additional workload. In essence, your muscles become stronger and denser and, as a result, better able to withstand stress in the future.

Here's an example of how you might progress in a strength-training program: Say that you're just getting started on a workout regimen and can perform ten repetitions of a barbell bench press using 100-pound weights. If you do four sets of this exercise three days a week (say Monday, Wednesday, and Friday), your muscles will become denser and stronger, and in two to three weeks you'll be able to do twelve to fourteen repetitions. At that point, you'll be ready to start lifting heavier weights (adding, say, five or ten pounds), so you should (temporarily) go back to doing just four sets of ten repetitions each and then gradually build up to fourteen or so repetitions. After a few more weeks, you'll be able to lift still-heavier weights.

This example illustrates the "progressive resistance" concept: as soon as your body adapts to lifting a heavier set of weights, you give it more. This process forces your muscles to acclimate and ultimately to become healthier, and it's a surefire way to build up your metabolism.

Why Blood Supply to Your Muscles Is So Important

As a practical matter, many different forms of exercise, including those that are designed primarily for aerobic conditioning, will generate some degree of strength and muscle development. But since strength-building exercises exert such formidable stresses, your muscles will need a greater supply of blood in order to carry on their restorative and strengthening processes.

Many of the strength-training principles I'll be teaching you are specifically designed to enhance the flow of blood to your muscles. When you are training properly, you'll notice a dramatic step-up in the amount of blood that rushes to your muscles. This is precisely what is supposed to happen—and will if you train correctly.

When blood is forced into your muscles during your weightlifting program, it helps speed up the process of repair which your muscle tissue needs to undergo. If you follow the program laid out in this book, your muscles will rebuild themselves, becoming denser and stronger than they were originally. That's why you must be careful and follow this program *to the letter*. Never perform your strength exercises out of order or train the same muscle group two days in a row. If you do, your muscles won't have sufficient time to repair themselves.

Before You Begin

Many people schedule their exercise routine close to mealtime. Don't do that! As mentioned above, one of the most important elements of weight training is that it forces huge amounts of blood to flow to your muscle tissue. This is what gives you the strength to do the exercise and enables your body to repair any temporary damage that may occur. Digestion is also a major user of blood, so subjecting your body to the processes of digestion and strenuous exercise simultaneously could cause your heart and your digestive system to be overworked, which could deprive your hungry muscles of the requisite nutrients.

If you program your exercise routine too close to mealtime, you'll end up compromising your strength-training program right from the start. Eating just after or just before your workout won't allow your system to get the proper amounts of blood it needs. Plan on waiting at least a full hour after a meal before exercising, and wait at least a half-hour after your workout is over before you eat your next meal.

Exercise Routine

When you're just beginning a weight-training program, it is important to limit yourself to exercises that are easy. A personal trainer can be a tremendous help in getting you started on the right foot. He or she is likely to recommend that you start with a one-set, ten-rep program of eight to ten different exercises that you're to do two or three times a week. (Don't be discouraged if you don't know what I mean by sets and reps. I explain these terms for you a little later in this chapter.)

Common exercises include the bench press, pull-downs, flies, bicep curls, incline sit-ups or leg lifts, squats, and a cardio routine. Whatever you do, be sure to tackle your chosen exercises in an appropriate order. There are many systematic ways in which you can train your muscles. I've included an example exercise routine in this book, but any qualified personal trainer or fitness coach can prescribe an exercise routine that's right for you.

Always train your muscle groups in an organized, systematic fashion. Typically, your trainer will recommend starting with a larger muscle group and working your way down to a smaller one. If you're doing more than one set of a particular exercise, you should complete all those sets before going on to the first set of another exercise. Moreover, you should do all the exercises for one muscle group before going on to another muscle group. Once you choose a predefined order in which to work your muscles, stick to it until and unless your trainer instructs you otherwise.

You will most likely be told to start by exercising your back, since this is your body's largest muscle group. Your back routine might include three sets of a rowing exercise. If this is the case, you should do all three sets, but allow a proper resting period in between, before moving on to the next exercise group.

And be sure not to do one set for your back, then one set for your arms, and then a repeat of the back exercise. Granted, at times it may not be so easy to fit in the various exercises in the proper exercise sequence, especially when your health club is extremely busy, but take your time and do it right.

If your back workout includes two or three different back exercises, then do all of those back exercises together before moving on to the exercises for some other muscle group (such as doing squats to strengthen your leg muscles). On a chest routine, you should do all of your bench presses first, then your incline bench presses, and finally your flies.

If you do your exercises "out of order," you'll miss the added benefit of fully targeting blood to just one muscle group at a time. Only by targeting your muscle power to one specific group at a time can you fully enjoy the stimulation that your exercise program provides and optimize the long-term benefits that you gain from it.

Simply stated, start with the largest muscle group, and finish exercising that group before moving on to the next-largest one. Then continue this process until you've completed your entire exercise routine.

The only note I would add is that your body will eventually get a bit "stale" as it becomes accustomed to your established exercise routine. This will probably happen about three months after you embark on your exercise program, provided that you've kept up with it on a regular basis during that time. To deal with this stale condition, you'll need to systematically alter the order in which you perform your exercises; otherwise, your results will begin to diminish. If you find that you need help with this, one thing you can do is to get hold of a good manual on exercise routines that will help you reach higher levels of success. (For example, you can order manuals on basic, intermediate, and advanced exercise programs either directly from my office or online via my Web site.)

Exercise Sets and Reps

Walk into any health club or gym, and you're bound to hear the terms *sets* and *reps*. A rep (which is short for "repetition") consists of a single performance of one particular weight-lifting or other exercise movement, while a set consists of the sum total of all the times that you engage in a particular movement in succession before taking a rest.

For example, suppose that you set out to do pushups. If you do just one pushup, that's one rep; if you do six pushups, that's six reps. If you then decide to stop and take a quick rest, even if it's just long enough to catch your breath, that signals the end of one set of pushups. If you then do six more reps (that is, after your short rest period), these six new pushups count as your second set.

The best way to increase your metabolism is to do three to four sets of eight to twelve reps apiece. For example, you might lift a certain weight eight to twelve times in succession, then rest for a bit (just long enough to allow your muscles to recover), and then repeat the entire cycle (of exercising and resting) two or three times. Typically, the breaks between sets would last about thirty seconds.

The number of sets per exercise is always a personal matter, and you'll notice that different exercisers are following different routines, according to their particular goals, interests, and personal preferences. One note here, and it's a very important one: Don't take the advice of other exercisers at a health club or gym. I'm sure they all mean well, but your goal is to persist in a given program, not to try one approach and then switch to another, helter-skelter.

It's best to take the advice of one source that you consider to be an expert. You can start by following the expert advice in this book. Once you've mastered every aspect of what's presented here, you should move on, either to a more advanced manual or to another fitness expert. Just be sure not to change your routine until you've truly mastered the one you're following at any given time; this is where so many otherwise-successful people fail miserably.

Progressive Resistance

As mentioned before, one of the wonderful things about muscles is that they get stronger and denser as we subject them to additional stress (in the form of progressively more-demanding exercises). That's why we must continually add more stress to our lifting program, by either increasing the amount of weight lifted or decreasing the duration of the rest period between sets.

As muscles adapt to a particular level of stress (weight or rest time), the amount of stress must be gently increased (by increasing the weight or cutting down on the rest period) if you are to continue to reap the benefits of the exercise in the form of denser, stronger muscles and an ever-increasing metabolism caused by those denser muscles. If you refrain from upping the level of stress, your program will still be beneficial, but you won't develop the muscle density that you've set your sights on.

Please remember that, as noted earlier, muscle *density* does not equate to muscle *size*. An increase in muscle density is a direct result of a rise in the concentration of muscle fibers that work in harmony within a particular muscle. In effect, the more compact and concentrated the muscle fibers, the stronger and more solid the muscle. An increase in muscle size, on the other hand, is achieved by performing a certain number of sets and reps of specific exercises in a way that increases not only the *density* of a muscle (the inner compactness of its fibers) but also its *volume*.

Progressive resistance is your key to muscle density and metabolic enhancement through anaerobic training. You may have heard progressive resistance referred to as "progressive overload." Same deal. No matter which term you use to describe it, this is just the periodic (and permanent) introduction of additional stress to an exercise routine, regardless of what form the added stress may take (either an increase in the "load" to which you subject your muscles in each set or a decrease in the duration of the rest period between sets).

By way of example, suppose your start your bench press by lifting 100-pound weights. In no time at all, you'll find that your arms, shoulders, and chest muscles have strengthened and become denser and that lifting 100 pounds is too easy. As a result, you'll have to either add weight or reduce the rest period between sets in order to prevent your muscles from becoming too comfortable. You can either move up in terms of the amount of weight lifted (say to 105 or 110 pounds) or decrease the rest period between sets (say from thirty seconds to twenty-five or even twenty seconds). As the weeks turn into months, you'll keep adding weight at a rate of about five pounds per month or decreasing the duration of the rest period between sets by five seconds per month. Once you reach a point where your rest period is down to only ten seconds between sets or you are unwilling to increase the amount of weight you're lifting, it's time to alter your exercise routine by choosing different exercises.

If your goals include increasing muscle size as well as muscle density, whether throughout your entire body or just in certain parts of your body, you can raise the amount of weight you lift in increments of ten pounds per month (rather than just five) without decreasing the rest period between sets. By making just that one modification, you will begin to add volume to your muscles.

To reiterate: if you want to continue to make progress, you must *progressively* increase the amount of weight you lift or decrease the length of the break between sets.

Another point you need to understand is that an increase in the number of reps will translate into an increase in strength. Some people believe they're capable of gaining strength only by increasing the amount of weight they lift. Not so! Strength can also be enhanced by increasing the number of reps. Muscular endurance comes from taking shorter breaks between sets, and muscular density/metabolic enhancement comes from persistently working on improving muscle strength and/or muscular endurance.

Always Exercise in Proper Form

You should always be sure to do your exercises in proper form. After all, the key to maximum metabolic benefit in strength-building exercises lies not just in *doing* an exercise (regardless of style or form). The essential ingredient is to do the exercises *correctly* so that you get the most out of each exercise you've chosen.

That's one of the reasons why health clubs usually have mirrors located near or around their free-weight area. The mirrors are there so that, among other things, you can pay particular attention to your form.

Your exercising motions should be clean and fluid and in a direct line with the muscle's proper axis. If at all possible, you should not allow your line of exercise motion to stray. Pay close attention to maintaining good form from the first rep of the first set to the last rep of the final set. Never jerk or throw the weights around. Never create an unbalanced movement (that is, you should never hold less weight in one hand than you hold in the other). Whenever possible, work out with a training partner, someone who can assist you in your workouts and whom you can assist in return.

Negative and Positive Resistance

Whenever you do any type of strength-training exercise, you're really asking two different parts of your muscle to participate. The "positive" phase of the exercise, which takes place while the muscle is lifting a weight (either lifting the dumbbell in a bicep curl or elevating the bar in a bench press), is called *concentric contraction*. The end of that motion is the point at which your arms are close to your chest (in the curl) or fully extended (in the case of the bench press).

The other part is the *eccentric contraction*, which is termed the "negative" phase of the exercise. This is the phase that calls upon muscle resistance as you slowly return the weight to its starting position.

Interestingly enough, it's just as important, if not more important and more physiologically demanding, to let the weight slowly return to the original position in the negative phase as it is to push or pull the weight, as the case may be, in the positive phase. Returning the weight slowly and with resistance on every repetition is important, because this is the phase that promotes greater flow of red blood cells to your muscles, which in turn builds greater strength.

Of course, another way you'll know your form is correct, in addition to using mirrors to check yourself as you exercise, is that you'll feel warmth, some fatigue, and a "burning" feeling at the end of each set for each muscle group. If you don't get this sensation, review your form and pay greater attention to what you see in the mirrors. They're telling you something. Your form may be poor, and if so, you may not be allowing a full complement of blood to reach your target muscles.

Though getting tired is not a sure sign that you're doing an exercise correctly, either feeling lactic acid accumulate in your muscles or not experiencing fatigue is usually is a sure sign that you're *not* doing it right.

Lifting Speed

In addition to lifting *form*, lifting *speed* is an important element that has a major effect on how much blood moves to your target muscles. And while you might think that the faster you lift the weights the sooner you'll notice great results, the opposite is true.

Although fast lifting creates a certain momentum, it doesn't promote optimal blood flow to the muscle. What does promote this blood flow is slower movement. Slow lifting creates less internal muscle friction and requires a more even application of your muscle power through your range of motion.

You say you don't believe me? Well, just try it. For example, try doing a bench press with a slow, even pressure, and be sure to do it with perfect form and no wavering. You'll find it's much more difficult than a quick pressing motion. The slower movement also generates a more rapid flow of blood to the muscle groups you are training. You might also unwittingly discover that too much speed has the undesirable effect of increasing your frequency of lifting-related injury.

Your exercise trainer might recommend, as I do, taking one to two seconds for each lifting movement (the positive phase) and three to four seconds for each lowering movement (the negative phase).

Whatever your actual lifting speed, always remember to come back slower during the resistance phase with each and every repetition. All of which brings us back to proper form. If you discover that the weight you've chosen to lift in a certain exercise is so heavy that you cannot maintain proper form and at the same time perform the negative phase slowly and in full control, you should lighten the weight until you can do it exactly as intended.

Far too many beginners pay attention only to the amount of the weight to be lifted, and not to the quality of the movement performed. Your muscles cannot know how much weight is on the bar or machine, but they will respond very well if you are not only using good, controlled form but also executing the return phase slowly and with the proper resistance.

Exercise Selection

It is very important to select at least one exercise for each major muscle group in order to promote well-balanced muscle development. Training only a few muscle groups, or training one particular muscle group more than the others, increases the risk of injury.

Exercise Sequence

Another important element of strength training is exercise sequence. When performing a variety of weightlifting exercises, it is advisable to proceed from the larger muscle groups to the smaller muscle groups. This allows for optimal performance of the most demanding exercises at those times when you are feeling fresh and energetic and your fatigue levels are at their lowest.

Another reason for starting with the larger muscle groups, one that is often overlooked, is illustrated by the common example of training both back and biceps. Ordinarily, you would want to train your back first, since it is the larger muscle group of the two. So let's say you're doing the Rear Pull-Down. In that exercise, you are indirectly working your biceps, too, since both muscle groups are at work in the pulling motion. This means that your biceps will actually be warmed up and ready to train when you get to exercises that focus directly on them.

You will derive a similar benefit when you perform exercises that require pushing motions, since they tend to involve use of the chest, shoulders, and triceps. By the time you're done with your chest exercises, both your shoulders and your triceps will be warm and ready to train. Of course, you might not always do your pulling motions (the ones with your back and biceps) on the same day as your pushing motions (the ones with your chest, shoulders, and triceps). In fact, as you advance you will want to split up your exercise days so that you train certain muscles on one day of the week and others on a different day. This topic will be discussed a little later.

To Avoid Injury, Avoid Over-Training

Beginning weight-trainers are often a gung-ho group. Unfortunately, that's one of the major reasons why so many of them drop out long before they've given themselves a chance to adjust to a healthful change in lifestyle.

Be sure to pay close attention to your body and to what it tries to tell you. If you ever find that you're feeling weak, sore, "burnt out," or wishing you could skip a workout, you may well be over-training. This is a common complaint of beginners.

Not providing your muscles with enough rest could very well hinder your progress. Training the wrong muscle groups on consecutive days—or doing too many sets or exercises on the same muscle group—may also set you on the road to failure. Remember, weightlifting temporarily "injures" the muscles that you're training, and they need time to recover and grow. Ordinarily, that rejuvenation process takes a couple of days, so the watchword is: don't exercise the same muscle group two days in a row.

As you become slightly more advanced in your exercise program, you may find that splitting up your training days is more effective for you. Suppose, for example, that you wish to adopt a weekly routine that includes chest, shoulders, triceps, and abdominal muscles (*abs* for short) on Monday. Then on Tuesday you might switch your routine and exercise your back, legs, biceps, and abdominals/stomach muscles. (Note that you can train your abs on both of those training days, but then be sure to give your whole body a needed rest on Wednesday—you deserve it!)

You could go back to the chest group, including chest, shoulders, triceps, and abdominal muscles, on Thursday. And on Friday you could again exercise your biceps, abs, legs, and back. Then you would rest over the weekend and start all over on Monday.

Whatever routine you create, remember one thing: Listen to your body! If you're over-training, your body will tell you. If that happens, take it easy. Allow your muscles to grow and strengthen at *their* pace, rather than according to some arbitrary schedule you've set up for yourself.

In no time at all, you'll begin achieving spectacular results. And I'm not talking just about the results you can *see*: the shapelier body; the smooth, sculptured muscles; the tight, toned physique. I'm talking about the high-speed metabolic system you've created that's constantly burning up calories each morning and afternoon, and even while you sleep. It's incredible, and so are the results you can obtain by undertaking the other important half of the metabolic-exercising duo: aerobic exercise.

10

Your Cardiovascular Metabolic Tune-up

Fitness That Forces Your Metabolism to Burn Hotter Than Hot

Now that I've introduced you to the metabolic underpinnings of my strength-training program, you're ready to get started on the logistics of a good cardiovascular program. Metabolic fitness includes both aerobic and strength-training elements, and they work together to produce total metabolic health.

As you learned in the previous chapter, aerobic exercises include that very large class of movements that can be performed only by burning huge amounts of oxygen. We're talking about running, jogging, spinning® (an aerobics class on bikes), power walking, cross-country skiing, etc. Since they place such heavy demands on your heart and lungs, it should come as no surprise that they are excellent exercises to promote cardiovascular fitness.

However, they also *burn calories*, and that's why they're so important when it comes to increasing your metabolism. Not only does aerobic exercise burn more calories *as* you exercise, it keeps your metabolic rate high for several hours *afterwards*!

We've seen that proper exercise, along with a good diet that's low in fat, moderate in carbohydrates, and high in protein, is crucial for metabolic control, because both dieting and exercise help reduce body fat. Moreover, exercise works in still other ways to promote weight loss.

Exercise Regulates Appetite

Appetite has to do with our *psychological* desire for food. *Hunger*, in contrast, refers to our *physiological* requirement for nutrition. In other words, appetite refers to the *food we crave*, while hunger refers to the *nutrition our bodies need.*

One belief that's widely held in America is that exercise increases appetite, leading to increased calorie consumption and the risk of weight gain. Actually, just the opposite is true. Regular exercise moderates the cravings that can lead to weight gain. With all those fad diets, we eat less because we *make* ourselves eat less—and this can actually increase our appetite. With exercise, we eat less because we *want* less.

This happens for well-documented physiological reasons that center on the hypothalamus, a gland that's located in the brain and exerts a specific type of control over our metabolic rate. Besides producing essential hormones, the hypothalamus triggers our sense of hunger. It is a commonly accepted theory that we feel hungry when the glucose supply to our brain gets too low. Sensing this, the hypothalamus sends out warnings of an impending food deficit. In response, we start thinking about food and our stomach contracts, leading to the sensation of "growling." Then our body secretes chemicals, such as hydrochloric acid, to help us digest the upcoming meal.

Exercise inhibits hunger by raising the levels of certain chemicals in the blood and brain: glucose, serotonin, noradrenaline, adrenaline, and dopamine. These chemicals send a signal to the brain to announce that the body's hunger has been satisfied. In effect, regular exercise leads us to say "I'm full" sooner than we would if we were not exercising regularly. What's more, this sense of reduced appetite may last for as long as six hours after we finish exercising.

Other researchers have pointed out that the exercising body is much more likely to *crave* the foods that are important for physical performance. Many people who exercise regularly are drawn to the more wholesome complex carbohydrates and proteins that the body needs to function well. Research suggests that exercisers lose weight because of the body's *natural* preference for good food and its aversion to fats and simple carbohydrates that inhibit athletic performance.

What does all this mean? Does it perhaps mean that the more we exercise, the less hungry we'll be? NO! It means that proper exercise inhibits hunger—to a point. But remember, we're building muscle density, and the denser the muscles, the more calories they will consume. If we don't supply them with FAT from our foods, they will burn the fat already stored in our body!!!

After all is said and done, we *may* be slightly hungrier as a result of exercising, but our body will crave foods that are more healthful and it will burn body fat for energy. And therein lies the magic!

Exercise Can Elevate Our Mood

Another contribution that exercise can make to the weight-loss process resides in its unique ability to alter mood. Depression, boredom, fatigue, and stress are very common complaints of Americans. Moreover, such complaints are quite prevalent among those who are overweight.

Mood swings can be problematic for anyone. Some people eat for the express purpose of filling an emotional void, or to ward off feelings of loneliness, boredom, or depression. It isn't hard at all to see how so many people with emotional disorders end up becoming compulsive overeaters. In effect, they use food to alter their mood, much like those who are addicted to mind-altering chemicals.

Exercise, in contrast, provides a calorie-free "high" that *dependably* helps us manage our moods and our weight. The results of research studies undertaken on a nationwide scale have shown that adults who are physically inactive are at much greater risk of feeling the effects of mood than those who regularly engage in physical activity.

Most individuals report that they experience an overall sense of wellness or feel energized following vigorous aerobic exercise. Countless studies show that depression, anxiety, and mood state are favorably affected by regular exercise, which can also help improve a person's self-esteem.

Getting Your Cardiovascular Training Program Started

The best way to start your program of aerobic fitness is to demonstrate some good, common sense and see your doctor. As perfunctory as this advice may seem, it's a great step to take—and for reasons far more important than the obvious.

First of all, a complete physical exam will yield important information about the condition of your heart. For example, The American College of Sports Medicine warns that people with a history of high blood pressure or abnormal resting EKGs, or a family history of heart disease, run a higher-than-average risk of causing injury to the heart as a result of performing certain exercises. Only your physician can provide the information you need to make an intelligent decision in this regard.

Also important is the feedback you'll get—if you ask for it—in the way of test results from your doctor's lab. The staff at any lab that's worth its salt will scrutinize your blood chemistry and give you important information that will enable you to track your fitness progress.

By knowing HDL and LDL cholesterol levels, for example, you can chart improvements in your body chemistry as you exercise. The same is true of the levels of triglycerides and glucose in your blood. Since these levels can be improved through exercise and diet, you'll gain solid evidence of how unseen chemical reactions in your body are improving through the use of this program.

Test Your Physiological Condition

Your next step is to find out what kind of physiological shape you're in. Again, this is recommended simply to help establish benchmarks regarding your present condition so that you can set reasonable expectations for the rate of progress you'll be making in the weeks and months ahead.

Any quality health club can provide a number of different tests that take only a few minutes each. These tests can show you how you stack up—in terms of key fitness components such as muscle strength, cardiovascular fitness, and flexibility—against others in your age group.

The beauty of these tests is that once you've taken them, you can intelligently set goals and chart your progress. You may, for example, wish to reduce your resting heart rate from its present 75 beats per minute to a new goal of 65. Or you might want to reduce your heart's recovery time. Every area of fitness that you succeed in improving will assist you in creating a more powerful metabolism and a healthier body.

A good health club will also help you set realistic goals for the future, whether you become a member or not.

Rating Cardiovascular Exercises

There are an almost-unending variety of exercises from which to choose when planning your aerobics program. Some can be done only in summer, others only in winter. Some are strictly indoor pursuits, while others are clearly outdoor activities. Some involve specialized equipment, while others can be done with little more than a good pair of shoes and a T-shirt.

In this book, we'll focus exclusively on those exercises that most easily lend themselves to some sort of objective measure of improvement in health and fitness. The easier it is to measure the number of calories expended, the easier it will be to predict the results you will realize from doing an exercise. This is one of the main reasons why I believe everyone should become a member of a good health club. Health clubs provide measurable results, whereas outdoor activities are harder to measure because of all of the external variables that tend to modify one's daily exercise program (wind direction, temperature, and precipitation, as well as factors such as the presence of cars, trucks, or other exercisers that get in the way while you're trying to jog or ride a bike).

Aerobic exercises

Aerobics classes are one example of a good total-body exercise. To get really dramatic results from this type of activity, however, people often go the high-impact-exercise route, where overuse injuries are common.

Running and jogging on a treadmill are also great exercises for cardiovascular conditioning. But again, they are high-impact exercises that frequently cause an undue amount of damage to the feet, ankles, legs, or hips. If done without regular stretching, these exercises can actually reduce flexibility. Proper use of a treadmill, however, considerably reduces your chances of injury, and it allows you to monitor your heart rate at the same time.

Indoor rowing (on a rowing machine) is one of the top-rated aerobic exercises.

Spinning® and indoor rock climbing are two of the best aerobic exercises you can choose—according to some studies, at least. They tend to be gentler on joints and bones than the high-impact exercises, and yet they aid in conditioning all the major upper- and lower-body muscle groups.

Walking on a treadmill has always been a popular exercise, but it needs to be done at a brisk, "power-walking" pace to get the full cardiovascular benefit. Most people don't walk fast enough, or at a high enough incline, to get an aerobic workout.

Exercising the MYM *(Maximize Your Metabolism)* Way

No matter what sort of exercise you choose, it should be incorporated into a proven system that maximizes aerobic effect and minimizes personal injury. The MYM formula was created after years of personal study and input from many major health and fitness associations such as the American College of Sports Medicine. It includes five crucial elements:

1. Aerobic warm-up
2. Minor stretching
3. Aerobic and strength conditioning
4. Aerobic cool-down
5. Final, more-detailed stretching

If at first glance this looks like a lot of exercise, don't let it overwhelm you. You have a choice of when to do both your aerobic and strength-conditioning workouts, either on the same day or on an alternating basis. Your warm-up, stretching, and cool-down sessions will be fairly brief, as explained below, but they do need to be part and parcel of every workout session.

The MYM *(Maximize Your Metabolism)* formula

1. The Warm-up. The first step in any exercise program is the warm-up. The purpose of the warm-up is to elevate the core temperature of your muscles, increase your pulse rate and the flow of blood throughout your body, and prepare your body for exercise. Your warm-up should be of low intensity, and it should last five to ten minutes. It might include brisk walking, performing jumping jacks, or doing some indoor cycling.

2. Stretching. The second component of an exercise program is stretching. Stretching the major muscles of the body prior to exercising prepares the body for the meat of your workout. Stretching helps to enhance your physical performance, prevents debilitating injuries, and makes you look and feel better by improving your muscle elasticity.

Proper stretching of the muscles will increase your range of motion and improve the quality of your movements. Never stretch a cold muscle! Always make sure your muscles are warmed up before you begin to stretch. When a muscle is properly warmed up, it is filled with healthy, oxygenated blood, which then circulates to nearby tissues and helps remove unwanted waste products from your system.

Be sure to pay special attention to the primary muscles you used in your warm-up. If you did your warm-up on a bicycle, for example, then it's okay to stretch all of your muscles, but pay special attention to the ones you used in the warm-up. (In the example of warming up on a bicycle, it would be your quadriceps, hamstrings, calves, and hips.)

When stretching, remember to adhere to the following guidelines:

- Stretch slowly and in a controlled manner, and assume a comfortable position (but never bounce)
- Stretch a muscle to the point of light tension, not pain
- Hold each stretch for fifteen to thirty seconds, then slowly release and return to the starting configuration
- Take slow, deep breaths while stretching, and do *not* hold your breath
- Increase the effort and duration of each stretch at regular intervals, to continue improving your flexibility
- Include stretches for the entire body
- To prevent boredom, learn two or three difference stretches for each area of the body

Here are some stretching exercises you should include in your workouts.

Chest and shoulders (pectorals and deltoids)

Stand and keep your knees slightly bent. Bring your arms behind your back, clasping your hands together. Slowly lift upward. If you are unable to bring your hands together, simply bring them back as far as you feel comfortable. As you become more flexible and feel like increasing the stretch, bend forward at your waist and raise your arms higher. Hold the stretch for fifteen to thirty seconds.

Upper back and shoulder (rhomboids and deltoids)

Stand and keep your knees slightly bent. Reach across the front of your body with your right hand, grasping your left elbow. Slowly pull your left elbow across your chin toward your right shoulder. You should feel slight tension on the outside of your left arm and shoulder. Hold the stretch for fifteen to thirty seconds. Repeat with your other arm.

Back of arm, upper and middle back, and shoulder (triceps, latissimus dorsi, and deltoids)

Stand and raise both arms above your head. Drop your left hand behind your head. With your right hand, reach down to your left elbow and pull your elbow toward your head. Hold the stretch for fifteen to thirty seconds. Repeat with your other arm.

Back and hips (obliques, erector spinae, and gluteus)

Sit on the floor and fully extend both legs. Bend your left leg and cross it over your right leg. Place your left foot on the floor, on the outer side of your right knee. Keeping your buttocks on the floor, turn your upper body to the left. Using your right elbow, press against the outside of your left thigh. Hold this position steady for fifteen to thirty seconds. Switch sides and repeat.

Back of thigh (hamstrings)

Stand erect, with both feet flat on the floor and close together. Slowly bend at the hips, lowering your hand to the floor while keeping your knees locked and straight. Be cautious, and move slowly on this stretch. When you feel a slight tension in your lower back or at the backs of your legs, stop lowering your body and hold that position. Taking slow, deep breaths, hold the stretch for fifteen to thirty seconds.

Front of thigh (quadriceps)

Stand near a wall or stationary object, and place your right hand on that object at shoulder level for support. Lift your left heel toward your buttocks, and grasp your foot with your left hand. Keeping your knee, hip, and ankle in the same vertical plane, slowly raise your foot, using your hand. You should feel this stretch all along the front of your thigh. When you feel a slight stretch in your leg, stop and hold the stretch for fifteen to thirty seconds. Switch legs and repeat.

3, 4. Aerobic Conditioning and Cool-down. The third component of the exercise program is aerobic exercise. Your normal aerobic session is meant to burn fat by increasing your internal temperature. There is, however, another important aspect of this, and that's the fourth component: the aerobic cool-down.

A healthy individual should engage in cardiovascular exercise at least three to five times a week, for a minimum of twenty to forty-five minutes per session, with an intensity that's between 60 and 80 percent of your maximum heart rate (max HR). Here, however, we're going to increase these numbers a bit, because we're looking for safe but fast results: you're going to focus on performing your aerobic workout five or six times per week, for thirty to 60 minutes per session, at a heart rate of 70 to 80 percent of your max.

Your heart rate should be monitored during your exercise routine, either by taking your pulse via your wrist or your neck or by using a heart-rate monitor. For this program, you should invest in a good heart-rate monitor. (This shouldn't cost you more than about $75.) People who are currently out of shape or just starting out should begin training at a somewhat lower intensity, probably between 60 and 70 percent of their max HR.

Every aerobic workout, whether performed by a novice or an advanced trainer, should be started gradually. Begin with a five-minute warm-up at a low intensity (at about 50 to 60 percent of your max HR), do your full aerobic workout, and then end with a five- to ten-minute cool-down (at the same low intensity of 50 to 60 percent of your max HR).

It's important that you understand and implement different methods of cardiovascular exercise in your program. For example, you can ride a stationary bike a few days per week, do a brisk walking routine on a treadmill another day, and spend yet another day using an elliptical machine at your health club.

It is critical that you be aware of the different options (including machines) that are available for cardiovascular exercises, so that you can overcome any plateaus you encounter and prevent boredom as well. You will eventually experience both of these outcomes (plateaus *and* boredom) if you continue to do the same exercise—and in the same training style—for more than sixty to ninety days. In order to keep on realizing the kinds of results you desire, you should always be on the lookout for ways to vary your exercises and use different types of equipment. Then when you reach a plateau, you can simply change your routine and implement a new method.

Let's now discuss the three different training methods that you should work into your cardiovascular exercise program.

Continuous training

The first method, which is the most common and traditional way of doing cardiovascular exercise, is called continuous training. This means that you do one form of cardiovascular exercise, such as riding a stationary bike, for the full duration of your exercise session. As a result, you use the large muscle groups continuously for the entire routine.

This is the method that I suggest you use in each of your training sessions, unless you are already very skilled or are working out under the tutelage of a highly skilled personal trainer. This is not to say that you shouldn't vary your exercises, but all of my studies indicate that people get far better results from sticking to one particular exercise during each of their workouts. If you want to choose a different cardiovascular exercise for the *next* day's workout, that's where variety can come into play.

The next method is good for those individuals who are already very experienced (people with more than one year of heavy aerobic training experience).

Interval training

Interval training is an intermediate method of cardiovascular training and thus should not be done by beginners. Interval training consists of repeated intervals of relatively low intensity, such as walking, interspersed with intervals of high intensity, such as running.

The "light" intervals should be undertaken at an intensity ranging from 50 to 70 percent of your max HR, while the "heavy" intervals should be done at an intensity ranging from 75 to 85 percent of your max HR (though you should get an okay by your physician before training at an intensity greater than 80 percent of your max HR). In either case (light or heavy interval), the intensity should be chosen on the basis of your functional capacity and your personal goals and interests.

The light intervals (in this example, walking) should take approximately thirty to sixty seconds to complete, and the heavy (running) intervals should last about one to two minutes. This form of training is prefaced with a two- to five-minute warm-up, and then the intervals begin. You should first do thirty seconds of light, followed immediately by one minute of heavy, then another thirty to sixty seconds of light, then one to two minutes of heavy. Each pair of intervals should be repeated only about fifteen times.

Please note: Before doing your interval training, warm up with one type of cardiovascular activity for about two to five minutes, then stretch the muscles that you used for that activity, and finally launch into your interval training.

If you're one of those people who are easily bored, you'll almost surely want to incorporate the next method into your program.

Composite training

The third training method, called composite training, is a combination of several different cardiovascular exercises, one after the other. One example is bicycling for ten minutes, then immediately switching to a treadmill for ten minutes, followed by running or jogging for ten minutes, then bicycling again or jumping onto an elliptical machine, and ending with a cool-down and stretching of the muscles used. Or you could walk on a treadmill for fifteen minutes, do the stair-climber for the next ten minutes, proceed to the elliptical machine, and then complete your thirty- to sixty-minute exercise period with a walking routine—followed, of course, by a cool-down and stretching session.

If you want to take it one step further and try something really intense and exciting, combine the interval training with the composite training. While you're on the treadmill, for example, you could either change the speed (from walking to jogging) or alter the inclination of the surface (from horizontal, say, to a 5-percent grade) every other minute. After ten minutes on the treadmill, you could move on to the stationary bike, changing the resistance from more intense to less intense every other minute.

Remember, you should always begin with a low-intensity warm-up and then stretch the muscles you used in that activity. You should conclude your workout with a cool-down of five to ten minutes (also at low intensity) and a stretch.

Measuring your heart rate

While following this program, I suggest monitoring your heart rate at all times in order to keep track of your intensity during any cardiovascular exercise. (Using a heart-rate monitor will make this much easier for you.) Exercise that does not raise your heart rate to a certain level—and keep it there for thirty minutes—WILL NOT contribute significantly to reaching your maximum metabolic rate.

The heart rate that you should maintain during exercise is called your target heart rate. There are several formulas for arriving at this figure. One of the simplest, which gives lower and upper bounds on the heart rate you should aim for, is as follows:

(220 minus your age) multiplied by 0.70 = your lower bound

(220 minus your age) multiplied by 0.80 = your upper bound

According to this formula, the target heart-rate range for a forty-year-old would be 126–144 (126 being the lower bound, and 144 the upper). What this means is that if forty-year-olds are exercising but their heart rate is below 126 beats per minute, then they aren't exercising as efficiently as they should be. If, on the other hand, their heart rate is over 144, then they're literally burning muscle rather than fat—and putting themselves at greater risk of heart injury during the exercise itself.

Some methods for figuring your target heart rate take individual differences into consideration. Here's a step-by-step formula you can use for that purpose:

1. Subtract your age from 220 to find your maximum heart rate
2. Subtract your resting heart rate (see below) from your maximum heart rate to determine your heart-rate reserve
3. Take 70 percent of your heart-rate reserve (multiply it by 0.70) to determine your heart-rate rise
4. Add your heart-rate rise to your resting heart rate to find your target rate

Resting heart rate should be determined by taking your pulse after sitting quietly for five minutes. When checking your heart rate during a workout, you should take your pulse within five seconds after interrupting your exercise routine, because the rate will start to go down once you stop moving. Count your pulse for six seconds, and multiply by ten to get the per-minute rate. If you have access to a personal trainer, be sure to ask him or her to do this for you; otherwise, you can take a reading of your heart-rate monitor, which will give you the most accurate count without your having to stop exercising.

When to exercise

The hour just before the evening meal is a popular time for exercise. A late-afternoon workout provides a welcome change of pace at the end of the workday and helps dissolve the day's worries and tensions.

Another popular time to work out is early morning, before the workday begins. Advocates of the early start say it makes them more alert and energetic on the job.

Among the factors you should consider in developing your workout schedule are personal preference, job and family responsibilities, and availability of exercise facilities. It's important to schedule your workouts for a time when there is little chance that you will have to cancel or interrupt them because of other demands on your time. (Metropolitan Life Insurance Company, 1996)

No more excuses, no more procrastination

During the next few months, you will probably come up with plenty of excuses as to why you should skip a workout or two. But keep in mind that the human mind can be trained to make a habit of something if that thing is performed for twenty-seven days in a row. Let's commit to making fitness a lifestyle, by not missing any scheduled workouts for the next twenty-eight or more days.

Remember, the key to staying motivated and continuing to achieve the results you want is to **keep your exercise program fun and exciting** by constantly trying new exercises.

5. Final Stretching. The fifth and final component of the MYM Fitness Formula is stretching. The same stretching exercises performed at the start of the workout can and should be performed again. In fact, it is during the stretching period after a workout that the majority of gains in flexibility occur. Stretching also aids in flushing the muscles of undesirable biochemical by-products of exercise, such as lactic acid, that can cause soreness.

Exercising Smart to Prevent Injuries

Despite the best-intentioned exercise plans, injury may occur. Undoubtedly, the best way to deal with injury is prevention. This is best accomplished with sensible training and a knowledgeable approach to your exercise routine. The following guidelines should help make your training both safe and enjoyable.

Golden rules of exercising

- Avoid strenuous exercise if you are feeling ill or have been sick for an extended period of time.
- Exercise with the proper frequency: three to five days per week of aerobic exercise, and three days per week (every other day) of strength-training exercise.
- Exercise at the intensity level that's best for your individual fitness needs.

  If you're just beginning an exercise program, exercise at a heart rate that's near the lower end of your target heart-rate range, and then gradually increase the intensity of your workouts.

- Always use proper form when exercising (never sacrifice form in order to lift heavier weights during a strength-training workout).
- Wear shoes that are designed for the exercise you're doing (running shoes for running, cross trainers for cross training, good walking shoes for dedicated walkers), and wear comfortable clothing (the kind that allows your body to sweat).

  If exercising outdoors, take weather conditions into account before you leave for your workout.

- Avoid doing any **one** exercise too often.

  Performing one exercise over and over can tire the muscles involved in that exercise and cause unnecessary muscle strain. Adding variety to your workout allows you to work your muscles differently and continue building your motivation.

- Drink plenty of water.

  Drinking water before, during, and after a workout is essential. From an exercise standpoint, replenishing your body's water supply greatly enhances your strength, speed, and endurance. Experts recommend drinking up to twenty ounces of water during the hour or two before you begin exercising, and taking another three to six ounces every ten minutes during your exercise period. I advise my clients to keep with them a sipper bottle filled with water while they're exercising, and to sip on it throughout the entire workout.

If You Are Injured

If you become injured, consult your personal physician immediately. If you choose not to see your physician, the "r.i.c.e." treatment is often best: **r**est, **i**ce, **c**ompression, **e**levation.

- **R**est the injured body part (for no less than forty-eight hours) to prevent further injury and to initiate the healing process.
- **I**ce the injured area immediately for fifteen to twenty **minutes**, and repeat three to four times a day, to help reduce internal bleeding and keep the swelling down.
- **C**ompression provided with semi-firm **bandaging** will keep the swelling down and provide comfort.
- **E**levate the injured area, to allow blood to drain **back** to the heart and prevent it from pooling in the injured area.

11

Oxygen Creates Movement Before Movement Creates Oxygen

Easy Breathing Exercises That Stimulate Your Metabolism and Cleanse Your Lymphatic System

Ultimately, everything we say about the metabolic system comes down to energy. Getting it. Storing it. Burning it. From a physiological standpoint, we quite literally have energy to burn. Our bodies can store tremendous reserves of all the enzymes, acids, and other important substances that enable our muscles to move and our metabolic systems to function at top efficiency. We have sufficient energy stores to enable us to exercise for five straight days without refueling. Even a couch potato has enough stored energy to provide for a 50-mile run.

The energy, of course, is stored as fat, and using these energy stores in a metabolically efficient manner is the real sticking point. That's why learning how to maximize your access to these fuels is a crucial step in your metabolic makeover. As you're well aware, this book has tried in many ways to impress you with the importance of proper fitness and nutrition. However, all the best exercises and all the best nutrition in the world will be useless unless your body has the proper amount of oxygen to unleash its energy. Oxygen is a crucial component to a strong and healthy metabolism.

There's Magic in the Air

You may not realize it, but your lungs aren't simply empty sacs that automatically inflate and deflate. They're organs crowded with specialized tissues designed for this crucial exchange of a variety of gases and the metabolism that follows.

Each of your lungs weighs about a pound. Since lungs do not have muscles, they depend on muscles in the rib and stomach areas for their crucial movements. Your diaphragm (that partition of muscle and connective tissue that separates the chest and abdominal cavities) contracts and flattens. At the same time, the muscles in the vicinity of your ribs gently pull the rib cage upward. This enlarges the chest cavity and causes air to be "sucked" into the lungs. When the rib muscles and diaphragm relax to their original positions, air is forced out.

On a day that's devoid of aerobic exercise, you'll unthinkingly perform this exchange about 20,000 times. Over an entire lifetime, that amounts to more than half a billion round trips. And it's all automatic: no thought, no preparation. Your medulla, that part of the brain stem that controls involuntary action, keeps all this equipment working without conscious thought. If it didn't, you'd die within minutes.

Your Air Exchange System

A breath of fresh air can enter your lungs through your nose or your mouth. As you probably learned in your high-school health class, the nose is the preferred route. The hairs in the nose help not only to filter the air of impurities but also to warm the air you breathe, bringing it closer to a temperature that your body can use effectively.

When you exercise vigorously, especially when you do aerobic exercises, you may start to pant. That's not because your lungs need more air; it's because your blood has too much carbon dioxide. The need for oxygen in your muscles is more than the heart can handle, forcing fuel to be burned with little or no oxygen—anaerobically. The result is a buildup of lactic acid, which causes muscle soreness and fatigue.

To neutralize this buildup, the body produces more carbon dioxide. The brain causes the breathing rate to quicken in order to raise the amount of oxygen coming in and, in turn, to increase the elimination of carbon dioxide. During a vigorous workout, you'll probably need more air than your nose will allow, so the overwhelming amount of respiration will take place through the mouth.

In either event, the diaphragm and the muscles in the rib area move to create the suction that draws air into the chest, expanding the lungs. In the lungs, tiny elastic balloons called alveoli process the air, and a gas exchange takes place. The oxygen from the inhaled air diffuses and saturates the hemoglobin in your red blood cells. Meanwhile, the blood, anxious to take on the oxygen, discharges carbon dioxide through the capillary walls into the alveoli.

The rest of the oxygen journey is fascinating, though it isn't vital that you know all about it in order to participate in the MYM program. If you're interested, I suggest picking up one of the many science books that lay out the full path in a far more detailed explanation than I will get into here.

Oxygen Becomes the All-Important Ingredient

The fuel that enables you to move your muscles is a chemical made by the body called adenosine triphosphate (ATP). This is the basic energy source for muscular contraction.

However, the body has only enough ATP on hand to fuel activity for about ten seconds. Once the store of ATP is used up, you've got to *manufacture* ATP. Your body can easily do that, but not without oxygen. When you engage in vigorous activity such as what we're recommending here, the body requires *lots* of oxygen. That's why I've devoted an entire chapter to teaching you how to get it more efficiently.

In order to speed up the metabolism, the body needs larger-than-normal supplies of oxygen, not only to manufacture ATP but also to accommodate the waste products that are given off in the ATP-making process. ATP is produced at a high rate from carbohydrate (glycogen) stores within the muscle, but the by-product is lactic acid. Your body must dispose of this lactic acid; otherwise, your muscles will become so fatigued that you may have to wrap up your exercise session prematurely.

Your oxygen delivery system is crucial to your full metabolic development, because it is the main provider of ATP in any exercise session that lasts more than about three minutes.

O-X-Y-G-E-N Spells Greater Metabolism

As you can readily see, true metabolic enhancement comes from an efficient interconnection of several key components. Peak metabolism is enabled, in part, by the development of strong, healthy muscles through weight training and aerobic exercise. An optimal exercise regimen, in turn, is dependent on a good supply of oxygen, to produce the ATP you so desperately need for a good workout.

So, let's start out right. Let's start getting greater amounts of that precious oxygen you need, so you can further turn your metabolism into a real fat burner. We'll start by discussing the breathing process. This presentation is a bit technical, but it contains information that you need to have.

How to Breathe

Most of us have been brought up in what I call the suck-in-your-gut style of breathing, in which you expand your chest with each breath. As a result, the upper chest takes over the chore of breathing. This can lead to the high blood pressure, racing heart, and shallow breathing that fuel many of our ills, including headaches, heart disease, and hot flashes.

Even worse, this is probably the least efficient way to get oxygen surging through the body, because it doesn't put enough air into the lower lungs, which is where the blood flow is richest—and oxygen-rich blood is what your metabolic system thrives on. The more blood that comes in contact with the oxygen, the greater the amount of oxygen that's delivered to the various parts of the body.

Are You Breathing Properly?

Here's a quick way to find out if you're breathing properly: Lie on your back with a book on your stomach. Now inhale. What happens to the book? Well, if you're breathing properly, the book will rise. The problem I find with most newcomers to my health clubs is that they simply expand their chests when they breathe, and the book goes *down*. The effect is even more noticeable if you ask them to take a series of *deep* breaths.

Expanding only your chest when you breathe means that your diaphragm is rising, which will squeeze your lungs and *limit their capacity*. If both your chest and your belly expand with each breath, your diaphragm will flatten as you inhale, allowing your lungs to inflate fully with oxygen. That means you're maximizing your oxygen-delivery system, which in turn maximizes the amount of energy that's available to be burned.

The best way to breathe is diaphragmatically: breathe through your nose, and concentrate on making *both* your chest and your stomach move—not just one or the other. This forces your lungs to take in more oxygen than they could ever accommodate if you took shallower breaths. Aim for five to seven breaths per minute while engaged in normal, everyday activity. Obviously, the number of breaths you take each minute while you're exercising will be somewhat higher. Breathing diaphragmatically may cause your breaths to get a bit shallower, and the frequency of breathing will definitely increase. In addition, the air you breathe will most likely come from your mouth rather than your nose.

Sometime when you're not exercising, try this technique: Focus on your breath without trying to manipulate it in any way. Then, with your mouth closed, inhale quietly through your nose as you silently count to four. After that, hold your breath and count to sixteen. Finally, exhale through your mouth and count to eight.

Work to make your breathing deeper, slower, and quieter. Your chest and your belly should expand like a balloon as you inhale.

Breathing for Maximum Metabolism

I heartily recommend that you embark on a regular program of breathing exercises, as outlined above. You don't need to lie on your back to do breathing exercises, so you can do them at any time and in any place you choose. Just concentrate on the proper motion with each breath. Do this repeatedly, and you'll develop neuromuscular patterns that will help you breathe correctly while you're exercising. Do your breathing exercises at least twice a day, ten times each session, and then work your way up to three times a day.

Whatever you do, don't look upon your breathing exercises as an insignificant component of your overall health and fitness program. Improper breathing has held back many a person from attaining their peak health level and their peak efficiency level, both at home and at work. Devoting a few minutes to training one's body to breathe properly can *greatly* improve one's health and promote a greater degree of success and happiness.

Remember, you can try this breathing exercise at any time of the day or night. Though it may be easier at first to do it lying down, you can also do it sitting, standing, walking, and so on. It's an excellent exercise to try before you get out of bed in the morning, or whenever you are anxious, tense, or low on energy, since it will help relax you and flood your brain and your muscles with oxygen-rich blood. Over time, it will help deepen your breathing and make it more natural.

Other Tips on Proper Breathing

Although it has not been scientifically proven that your lungs can be improved through training, you can learn to use them more effectively. Here are a few ways you can do so:

Take deep breaths before you attempt to do anything that requires a great deal of physical exertion. As you approach a difficult exercise, for example, take five deep breaths. This will flush carbon dioxide from your bloodstream, so that even if the subsequent strenuous activity causes your blood to become saturated with carbon dioxide, it won't affect you all that much, not with all that oxygen in your bloodstream. Remember, shortness of breath isn't caused by the need of your lungs for oxygen, but by the excess of carbon dioxide in your blood.

Abdominal conditioning, such as sit-ups and crunches (sit-ups with your feet raised up on a chair or bed), can be helpful. However, the best approach is to give these muscles regular training, as outlined in the final chapter.

The Training Effect

The more you exercise, the better this whole oxygen-handling system works. What I've found with my clients is that well-trained runners accumulate less lactic acid than occasional joggers because they have higher anaerobic thresholds. This means their heart and blood vessels perform the gas exchange more efficiently, staving off the production of lactic acid. Remember, it's the accumulation of the poisonous lactic acid that shuts your exercising system down. Conversely, the more oxygen you take in, the harder your muscles can work, the greater their growth and development, and, ultimately, the faster and more efficient your metabolism becomes.

The training program outlined in this book will help to increase the capacity of your muscle fibers to extract oxygen from the blood, thereby enabling you to exercise more intensely before becoming short of breath.

Practice breathing properly, especially during your workouts. Take several deep breaths when you're weight training, just prior to lifting the weights. Always exhale during the negative phase of the exercise.

Proper breathing can help you in other ways as well

Helps counter stress. Just three to five deep, full breaths can transport you from panic to calmness by allowing extra oxygen into your brain and lower lungs, making you better able to focus.

Lessens headaches. The brain is a muscle, and as such requires a clean, fresh supply of oxygen-rich blood at all times. Without an adequate supply of blood, the brain cannot function properly. One of the signs of a lack of oxygen in the brain is a headache.

Helps reduce high blood pressure. Deep breathing can reduce stress, and stress is one of the major causes of heart disease. The *Journal of Human Hypertension* recently reported that just two ten-minute sessions of deep, slow breathing can lower the blood pressure by as much as eleven points.

Reduces menopausal hot flashes. According to a study reported in the medical journal *Menopause*, increasing the depth of your breaths while cutting your breathing rate in half (six to eight breaths per minute, instead of the usual fourteen to sixteen) can reduce the incidence of menopausal hot flashes.

Slows the aging process. As mentioned in other parts of this book, the body has a way of slowing down when you get older. By following this program, however, you'll help to stem this inexorable slide. According to some experts, if you don't practice deep breathing at least twice a day, your lung capacity at age seventy will be a third of what it was when you were twenty.

In summary, the way deep breathing works is that it leads to much greater intake of oxygen, meaning that the heart doesn't have to work so hard, ultimately bringing about a decrease in heart rate and blood pressure and enabling the entire body to enjoy an oxygen "bath." More oxygen translates into better digestion; better workouts; more energy; less stress; a longer, leaner, more attractive life; and a stronger metabolism!

12

Mastering Your Emotions and Your State of Mind

Discover How Your Emotional States Control Your Metabolism

"It has been my experience that people who successfully fit a healthful-living program into their lives rank being fit right up there with oxygen."

—Christopher V. Guerriero

Nothing of any value ever happens in life without there first being an intense desire for its achievement followed by a rigorous program of emotional management that keeps you focused on your goal. In the case of setting out to improve your health and fitness, your program of emotional management must enhance your metabolic function as well. Managing your emotions and feelings is critically important to successfully maximizing your metabolism and should be taken very seriously.

Emotions are the key to our hormonal responses. If we are in a depressed state (meaning that every time we think about our body, we think negative thoughts), then our hormones, glands, and related systems will all work in concert to keep us in a depressed state—an emotional state that in turn brings about a depressed or slower-working metabolism.

Fortunately, the opposite is also true! A heightened enthusiasm for life results in a heightened metabolism. As a matter of fact, whenever we enlist any negative emotions such as depression, anger, hatred, or jealousy, we slow the process of building our metabolism. More importantly, whenever we enlist positive emotions such as love, enthusiasm, or faith, we immediately strengthen the metabolism-building process. The upshot of this is that a positive emotional state can be very exciting—even monumental—if it's structured properly.

Mood and Food

You're probably already very familiar with how food alters mood. There are many people who have learned to deal with their emotions, whether positive or negative, by using food as a coping mechanism.

When they're happy, they eat. When they're depressed, they eat. When they're angry, they eat. When they're excited, they eat. After they feed their emotions with food, they may also feel guilty, so what happens then? You guessed it! They eat all the more, and the cycle starts all over.

Other people, because of chemical imbalances or emotional issues, have a difficult time eating normally. Sometimes they're able to exert considerable control over the types and quantity of food they eat, while at other times they may binge uncontrollably. The bottom line is that, much of the time, they're terribly preoccupied with food—and their relationship with food makes them miserable.

Hormonal Effects

Not only does food alter mood, but mood then proceeds to alter metabolism. We're all familiar with the phenomenon of wintertime weight gain. One of the reasons why that occurs is that we force our metabolism to slow down in winter: we sleep more, we're less energetic, and we're more prone to sadness and depression. As a result, our metabolism follows our mood on its downhill slide.

Much of this change is due to hormonal changes. It was this discovery that first led researchers to study the link between emotions, hormones, and metabolism.

What Is a Hormone?

In the simplest of terms, hormones are the "messengers" that your body uses to communicate with other tissues, using your bloodstream as a chemical freeway.

We could say that your brain acts as the traffic cop in this scenario. It directs hormones to various parts of your body and regulates the functioning of your cells. Hormones ultimately determine how you feel, both physically and emotionally.

You're probably familiar with some hormones, such as thyroid, insulin, testosterone, and estrogen. Each type of hormone performs a very unique role in the body and supports a wide range of physical functions. In order for the body to function optimally, all of our hormones must pull together and work as a team. And that means that they cannot be disrupted by the myriad of negative emotions that often come into play in our lives.

Changes in hormone levels can exert a profound influence on the amount of fat your metabolic system decides to store, as well as on a variety of other functions, including sexual desire, mood states, energy levels, and physical appearance (skin and muscle tone). Hormonal imbalances have also been closely associated with heart disease, osteoporosis, and certain types of cancer.

In short, because hormones impact your metabolic system and virtually every other major system and organ in the body, optimization of your emotions becomes a critical component in maximizing your metabolism. If you succeed on the emotional front, you're certain to end up looking, feeling, and performing at your best.

Managing Your Emotions

A big part of achieving metabolic success is learning to manage our emotions. All too often, we accept negative emotions as a "necessary evil" in our lives, something that we are powerless to control.

Nothing could be further from the truth. Though we all have "hot buttons" that can lead us to feel anxiety, anger, depression, or even burnout, we can learn to be sensitive to our emotions and take active steps to turn them all into metabolic enhancers.

The key is to become acutely aware of our emotions, and then learn how to develop alternative responses that turn undesirable situations into positive ones.

Managing Emotions: A Three-Pronged Program

People who lead high-stress lives need to develop a personal program of emotional management. Emotional management helps keep life's hassles in perspective and allows you to increase both your productivity and your performance in all areas of your life. A good emotional management program consists of three parts: physical fitness, effective time management, and self-image development.

Physical Fitness

By far the most important component of any emotional management program is an ongoing exercise program. Being physically fit pays handsome dividends to those who seek and demand personal excellence. This is because of exercise's unique ability to almost "inoculate" a person with a certain degree of immunity to stress.

Exercise is very effective in reducing anxiety, although precisely how this occurs is not fully understood. Some researchers believe exercise satisfies the evolutionary need of humans to engage in large-muscle, physically aggressive activity. Primitive humans frequently practiced this form of adaptive behavior, but in our sedentary, civilized lifestyle there are fewer outlets for behavior of this sort.

Certainly, one of the benefits of exercise, and perhaps one often overlooked by medical researchers, is that exercise takes one's mind off of the event that produced the negative emotion in the first place. Exercisers report that it's extremely difficult to concentrate on the negative event while participating in an intense workout.

My own research with my clients has shown that the physiological response of fit people to life's stressors is superior to that of the unfit. For example, several studies have shown that people with low levels of aerobic fitness experience greater cardiovascular stress than people with higher levels of fitness. The heart rates of the less-fit test subjects increased by nearly thirty beats per minute more than the heart rates of highly fit subjects when faced with a stressor.

Another study showed that physically fit subjects had significantly reduced psychosocial stress responses to various stressors as compared to their less-physically-fit counterparts. In plain language, what this says is that physically fit people perform better, both physiologically and psychologically, when faced with stressful situations—and it is in stressful situations that true excellence tends to be manifested. Moreover, some studies have demonstrated that fitness plays a vital role in the ability to recover from stressful events, both mental and physical.

According to the results of several recent experiments, the great stressors of life, such as those measured in the Holmes Stress Test, simply don't seem to impact the lives of physically fit people the way they do the unfit. A four-year study of corporate managers showed, for example, that physical fitness seemed to buffer the impact of the typical ill effects caused by stress.

Many other studies confirm these results, suggesting that being physically fit reduces the effects of stress. Similar outcomes have been reported among those who regularly engage in exercise, whether they are super physically fit or not. In practical terms, this means that regular exercise is like a soothing tonic that can be taken to produce results that are almost immediate as well as to provide long-term immunity to stress.

Endorphins: The Body's Natural Stress Relievers

Perhaps the best explanation as to precisely how exercise helps you manage your emotions—helps, that is, by reducing stress, tension, and anxiety and by enhancing self-awareness—has been put forth by biochemists. As found in numerous studies, the pituitary gland increases its production of endorphins during exercise. Endorphins have long been associated with pain reduction. Moreover, the endorphin level rises sharply during exercise, and is now believed to be responsible for the exercise-induced euphoria reported by many athletes and other exercisers.

Studies at Duke University Medical Center showed that exercise is associated with a significant reduction in negative emotional states, and with a significant increase in positive mood states such as a sense of vigor and self-appreciation.

Exercising to Reduce Stress

A program of regular cardiovascular exercise is a key component of emotional management. Research has found that the exercises most effective in reducing stress and enhancing mood are the same ones that produce the greatest levels of cardiovascular (aerobic) endurance.

Recommended exercises include riding a stationary bike, participating in an aerobics class or a group exercise class, or using weights in an aerobic fashion. Whatever the exercise, it should be vigorous enough to keep your heart rate in your target heart-rate range (as detailed earlier in this book).

The benefits of exercising to reduce stress are both immediate and long range. Not only can a proper exercise routine reduce the crush of stress *right now*, but it can also condition your body to handle stress better in the near future. And it doesn't take long for exercise to have this effect.

Your emotions are not always under your direct control, but your actions are.

It is extremely difficult, perhaps even impossible, to maintain a negative, metabolism-robbing emotion when your actions are in opposition to that emotion.

If you're feeling sad, for example, you often unwittingly enhance that emotion by adopting body language that supports sadness: shrugging your shoulders, hanging your head, and speaking in low, hushed tones.

However, did you know that you can help banish ALL negative emotion by adopting a physical presence and manner that's just the opposite of the emotion you're trying to eliminate? If you hold your head high, walk firmly upright with confidence and speed, and speak in an excited tone, in no time at all you'll discover that that negative emotion slips away as your new behavior creates an entirely new mindset. What's more, your metabolic rate will follow suit. The more positive your emotional level becomes, the greater the likelihood of your metabolism regaining its normal—or a slightly elevated—state.

Try it and see for yourself. It works every time.

Take Action

One piece of good news is that we can take ACTION to modify our emotions. For the same reasons that it's difficult to maintain a negative emotion when your body language is positive, it's also difficult to maintain a negative emotion when your *actions* are positive.

If you start to feel any negative symptoms, you should take immediate corrective action. Plan an activity which is the opposite of the emotion you're experiencing. Feeling down? Go to a concert. Take your child or a niece or nephew to the zoo or to a children's museum. Volunteer for a cause you believe in. Take up a new hobby, whether it's a simple one like gardening or a more demanding one like sailing, mountain climbing, or bungee jumping. Try a new exercise regimen. Get out and meet new people, and learn new things.

No matter what form it takes, becoming active and involved will give you a fresh view of what your life is about, enable you to learn new skills and techniques, and recharge your batteries. This not only builds good, positive emotions; it also alleviates boredom, reinvigorates your work ethic, and reminds you of the good you can actually accomplish.

Do One Thing at a Time

Another aid in managing your emotions is to concentrate on your immediate task. Clear the desk and your head, and let tomorrow's job wait. It also helps to do the most difficult tasks during your high-energy periods. You may want to map your daily energy to determine your peak hours. Keep track of the high-energy times of your day over a period of several weeks, look for patterns, and then de-stress accordingly.

Avoid Perfectionism

Thinking that a job has to be done perfectly is a setup for becoming overstressed. When you're overstressed, your performance levels decline—and that's exactly the opposite of what you want. Another trait that often accompanies perfectionism is procrastination. If we tell ourselves a job has to be done perfectly, we often put off doing it. That produces even greater stress and, ultimately, a vicious circle of defeat.

Stop Trying to Control Others

Worrying about things over which we have no control is a fruitless and unrewarding mode of behavior. Remember Reinhold Niebuhr's Serenity Prayer:

Accept the things we cannot change,
change the things we can,
and have the wisdom to know the difference.

Plan Playtime into Each Day

Make a point of setting aside some time for play, and then honor that commitment to yourself. What playtime consists of is different for different people. For purposes of improving your health and fitness, it would be best to plan "active" play into each day (over and above your exercise time). An example might be running around with your dog, playing a ten-minute game of basketball, or taking a walk around the lake or through the park on your lunch break.

Employers learned long ago that workers are more productive when they take short breaks twice a day. A good option for desk workers would be to take a nice, brisk walk on their work break, whether around the block or up and down the hallways. The important thing is to build breaks into our day as a matter of course. Whenever we avail ourselves of a chance to relax or to take a break, we greatly minimize the negative effects of both mental and physical stress.

In the end, it is you who are in charge of your emotions. And though you cannot gain control of every single event in your life, you can control your actions and your emotions and make them both positive and constructive. Adopting the measures we've discussed here will put you in charge of your life—and of your metabolism.

So let's sum up this chapter . . . . You cannot **Maximize Your Metabolism** without shutting out negative or depressing thoughts from your mind AND replacing them with positive, exciting thoughts that are powerful enough to alter your emotions and your actions. Speak positively to everyone you meet, think only positive thoughts, and train yourself to move about at double your usual speed.

Do this, starting today. I know it will be frustrating at first, but hold onto the notion that you're not doing this to benefit the people you're dealing with. Rather, you're doing it for a strictly selfish reason: to heighten your own metabolism.

13

Cut Years off of Your Efforts

Model the Behavior of Successful People

"Every successful person has at least one good lesson to teach. Learn by other people's mistakes!"

—Christopher V. Guerriero

Most attempts to change unwanted behavior fail. Even in the most successful clinical weight-loss programs, most patients who succeed in losing 10 percent of their body weight gain back two-thirds of that weight in a year—and end up gaining all of it back in five years.

The task of modifying one's behavior, however, is neither impossible nor hopeless. Our research has consistently shown that one way the overweight and those who lead sedentary lifestyles can mend their ways is to model their behavior after an approach taken by someone who has already successfully made a change in the desired direction. One of the most valuable aspects of this book—and I hope you use it this way—is that it can be followed as if the advice contained in it were being given to you by your personal mentor. I've mentored many people in my life, and perhaps the most surprising (indeed flattering!) trait I've seen in each of my successful clients/students/friends is their willingness to adopt most, if not all, of what I do and to follow my lead in aspects of their life that pertain to health and fitness.

As pointed out in an earlier part of this book, I've spent years distilling all of the successful methods I've encountered over the years. With the help of many clients, I've tested these methods to ensure that the results people obtained in their quest for better health and fitness could be duplicated. Finally, I've documented them in this book.

Until you find models of your own, I suggest using this book as your mentor. Keep it in your private library for repeated reference, and make sure that whomever you choose as a mentor understands everything that's outlined herein.

When you model the behavior of a successful person, you learn from their accomplishments as well as their mistakes. You can then proceed to build upon their accomplishments and avoid all the pitfalls that they encountered, thereby cutting years off of your efforts!

Let's face it, changing our behavior is often a lonely business. Oftentimes, when we look for support we can't find it, even—perhaps especially—from family members. In fact, family members often turn out to be far more of a hindrance than a help.

One study showed that the majority of survey respondents (74 percent) believed their mate was more likely to hinder their progress than to help. When queried about specific nonsupportive types of behavior, the respondents were sweepingly disheartened:

- 78 percent claimed that their partner snacked in front of them, despite the partner's realization that observing the snacking behavior made it more difficult for them to stick to their healthful diet
- 47 percent said their partner insulted them about their physical faults
- 70 percent felt that their partner "didn't seem to care" whether they were in shape or not

What About *Active* Support?

A remarkable 81 percent of partners "rarely compliment" them on their achievements.

If you can't get support at home, then where *can* you get the help you need to fully utilize the techniques outlined in this book? Well, there are two answers to this question. First, you can buddy up with someone. Give a willing friend a copy of this book, and ask them to read it concurrently with you. Then, after reading it through once, review each chapter together and hold each other accountable for following everything in that chapter. The second answer is to find someone who has successfully done what you want to do and model your behavior after their winning ways.

There are two possible pitfalls, however, that you should beware of:

First, you shouldn't set out to model the behavior of someone who has *just recently* lost a ton of weight, gained ten pounds of muscle, or adopted a healthful lifestyle. People like that have not yet had time to demonstrate long-term success; they have only just begun. Although getting on track is your first goal—and these would-be mentors may have your best interests at heart in trying to help you get there—your main goal is to reach your intended weight and then remain there by mastering your metabolism. You shouldn't get stuck on emulating the behavior of someone who has yet to prove their perseverance over the long haul.

Second, when people know that you're using them as a role model or a mentor, they tend to act like an expert and may offer their input to too great an extent, or in areas you don't want help in.

There are several ways to handle the mentoring of a person who wants to help you but may not know where to draw the line. My suggestion is to silently observe them. Don't let them in on your plan to use them as a role model. Just watch and interact with them. Feed off their energy, but use what you're learning here as your bible, so that you can identify their shortcomings and avoid following suit. But by all means, don't hesitate to absorb all of their positive traits.

You can also build your own fictitious mentoring group. This process may seem foolish, but it has helped hundreds of my clients reach their goals when they didn't have a coach to help them, or when I was already too booked up with personal clients to take on any more.

To build your group, simply go to someplace that's quiet and mentally build a group of four or five "fictitious" people (it usually helps to have both men and women in the group). Give each of the members of your fictitious group a distinct personality that will help you reach your goals.

For example, one member may have reached his/her goal weight years ago and may still look incredible. That person is the one who should tell you what you can expect and how to avoid all the pitfalls you may encounter along the way. Such a person may also be a bit more critical of you, and may try to get you to reach beyond your goals—simply because *they* did it, *they* succeeded in keeping off their excess weight. Give personalities to each of the members of your fictitious group, and *make them all very positive thinkers who use only helpful motivational advice to guide you.*

Now that you have your fictitious mentoring group, you must set up regular meetings with them. Never show up late for a meeting, and they'll never let you down. They'll always be there if you need to have an emergency meeting before you go out to eat with your friends, or if your spouse has just prepared a big, greasy meal for dinner and there's nothing healthful for you to eat.

Use your group to give you all the positive support you need, and *never* tell anyone else about your group.

The fictitious mentoring group is one of the most powerful health and fitness techniques ever studied. Use it wisely and often, and you'll soon see why so many people can attribute their success to this process. If you have family members or friends who are well informed about weight loss and the role that metabolism plays in it and are clearly supportive in helping you achieve your goals, use them as well.

D.R. Black demonstrated that couples lost significantly more weight than individual participants in a controlled weight-loss study (*Health Psychology*, 1990, 9:330–347). A study by J.B. Lassner showed similar results: behavior-change programs based on a family systems approach were more successful than programs without such support (*Annals of Behavioral Medicine*, 1991, 13:66–72). A common conclusion among studies of this type is that enhanced social support improves one's chances of long-term maintenance of weight loss.

Modeling Made Easy

A role model is a person you admire and whose behavior you want to emulate. The most important trait you should be looking for in a role model is successful achievement of what you wish to achieve.

This is true in any endeavor you might choose, not just in taking up a diet and exercise program. If you want to be more successful in your work, for example, seek out a person who's already successfully doing the type of work you do, and learn from that person's successes—and, yes, even from their failures.

It makes no sense whatsoever for you to bumble and stumble along, learning a new mode of behavior, when there's an ample supply of successful others out there who may be eager to share the secrets of their accomplishments with you. When you find such a person, learn as much as you can about how they achieved their goals, and learn to read into each person, so you'll be able to distinguish between when they're just bragging and when they're actually telling you what made them successful.

Role-Model Checklist

How much do you know about the person you admire most? His or her success is probably the most obvious trait that you've noticed, but that one attribute may not prove to be sufficient. Besides having already achieved what you are setting out to achieve, a role model should have the following qualities:

honesty
commitment
sense of humor
determination
good self-image
high moral values

Things to review and do

1. Describe the characteristics of the person you wish to model.
2. Do some research on where you'll most likely find such a mentor.
3. Begin looking for the kind of mentor you have in mind.

Keeping Company with Other Successful Individuals

When you keep company with winners in your pursuit of increased metabolism, some of their desire to achieve will rub off on you. That's one of the reasons given by dieting clubs such as Weight Watchers and Overeaters Anonymous for the higher rates of permanent weight loss among their members than among dieters who try to go it alone. Let's face it, getting in shape can be a lonely and difficult business. All too often, the dieter gets little or no help from his or her family and friends. I realize that these people want to help, but frankly, they most likely don't know *how* to support your efforts to change.

To improve your chances of success, seek out supportive friends who share your desire to rid themselves of unwanted behavior. Share this book with them, and begin living in a new, more healthful way.

Books That Offer Models

Just as you can learn to model your behavior after that of others with whom you associate, you can do the same thing by *reading* about the successful exploits of others.

You'd be surprised at how many others have tried and succeeded at doing precisely what you want to do. Some of them have gone on to write books about their trials, travails, and eventual achievement. Let me point out some of the books I'd recommend as being useful as you attempt to build up your enthusiasm and a strong will.

One such book is *Psycho-Cybernetics*, by Maxwell Maltz. This perennial bestseller has helped thousands of people just like you improve their lives through a remarkable program of exercises, many of which entail modeling the behavior of others who have been successful. Maltz suggests that you seek out these people, observe their behavior, and then imagine yourself performing in the same successful way.

Still another book which is excellent reading is Napoleon Hill's *Think and Grow Rich.* This upbeat work will teach you how to take a new look at yourself and will give you a realistic way to achieve your goals, whatever they may be. Hill was one of the first of the popular psychologists to recommend that you join what he calls a "master-mind group," a body of specially selected people who have the same goal in mind. Hill also recommends that you pattern your behavior after group participants that you have specially selected for the successes you wish to emulate. Hill's book is mainly focused on building wealth, but the techniques he uses are powerful, and they can easily be converted and used to help people get into great physical shape.

You might also choose any one of a number of good biographies about outstanding men and women whose salutary qualities you would do well to emulate. Contemporary mentors who have achieved greatness in their area of expertise, such as Lee Iacocca, Oprah Winfrey, Ted Turner, and Sandra Day O'Connor, provide excellent modeling support. There is something special in reading about the success of others that strengthens one's will to achieve. Reading, and the images it creates, can awaken the vast inner energy within you, which may have long been dormant and just waiting for such a revival.

I'm sure you'll find many other books that will inspire you in your quest for better health and fitness. Why not go to your library today and choose a couple of these books for your nightly reading project for the next thirty days? Books like these will be tremendously effective in helping you switch to your new mode of behavior. Your goal should include reading at least one autobiography of a successful person, or one book on mental training or self-improvement, each month.

What's a Dieter to Do?

In the course of this program, you can take several steps to improve your social support system for your weight-loss efforts and increase your chances of success.

First, make plans to solicit social support from *outside* the family. Help of this sort can come from many different sources—books, mentors, friends, or your own fictitious mentoring group, just to name a few.

Second, proactively enlist the help of your family. Include your mate if you believe he or she can provide positive support for you.

When one member of a family is not living healthfully or is physically unfit, that sends a ripple effect through the entire family unit. The other side of the family-influence coin is that every member of the family can eventually share in the benefits of a proper diet and fitness regimen. Just make sure, as stated earlier, that you first start the ball rolling by yourself. First, read this book from cover to cover, and then reread it one chapter at a time, putting the various dieting, exercise, and emotional management techniques into effect as you go. Next, start your visualization program (which will be explained in detail in chapter 14). Then, begin your mentoring program. Finally, invite your family to share in your new energy and enthusiasm toward your diet.

Third, *get active*! Ask for the help you need but are not getting. It will do absolute wonders for your motivation and self-confidence. Invite compliments, ask for greater help with your challenges, and solicit your partner's cooperation in your dieting or fitness regimen. At the very minimum, convince your partner to do his/her snacking in private.

Bear in mind that role models can motivate, but only if they are people whose achievements we find attainable. Comparing ourselves or our loved ones to superachievers won't shame us into performing better. It will simply leave us feeling worse.

14

Mind–Body Link and Laser Visualization

Your Body Is a Direct Reflection of the Way You See Yourself When You Close Your Eyes!

Change How You See Yourself, and You'll Change How Others See You!

Success, in the minds of many people, is an outside force that controls the direction of their lives. They believe in the outdated idea that "as the twig is bent, so grows the tree." In fact, they believe so strongly in that old adage that they grow up to lead lives that are governed by their past. They falsely harbor thoughts and feelings to the effect that dramatic change and self-improvement are impossible goals.

Unfortunately, until some awesome crisis causes them to confront their mistaken notion of reality and they actually accept responsibility for their fate, they'll continue to float through life being mere passengers on a ship of fate that's steered by others and by "luck." Their lifestyle will continue to be one of groping and coping, or of just "getting by." Such a lifestyle and thought pattern will take over every aspect of their lives, from their health to their appearance, from their fitness level to their finances, and will even paralyze them in their relationships.

The reality is that all of us can take charge of our lives and shape our destinies through a planned program of visualization exercises that can truly make us winners in all departments of life: in our physical health, our careers, our family relationships, our friendships, and virtually every other aspect as well.

I like to refer to this higher plane of living as being in a state of *Laser Visualization*, meaning that you have practiced and honed your ability to visualize the present and your desired future to such a degree that you can see it without ever closing your eyes. It means you can see the world around you, not as others see it, but rather as you have determined that you want it to look. It's all a matter of your outlook on life.

We all know that when we are depressed, nothing we do seems to go right. What usually triggers depression? Depression is triggered by the way we react to a certain person or event, such as a rainy day. If you tended to get depressed and sleepy when you were younger simply because it was a rainy day, then you probably still get sleepy and depressed whenever it rains.

Did you know there are people who actually get excited when it rains? What about all those kids who grow up loving to play in the rain? What kinds of feelings do you think *they* associate with rainy days? Let me tell you, rainy days are playtimes for them.

The moral of this story is that the rain does not determine your feelings, nor does it determine how you will act that day. You are in control of your every mood, and of every reaction you have to events and other people.

Let's look at another example that may be closer to home for you. Think of someone you really love (or someone you're really intimidated by—either scenario will work here). If you're in a bad mood, thinking about someone you truly love has a tendency to bring you right out of that mood. If you're in a great mood but you're told that you have to make a presentation to your intimidating boss, you might click into a depressed or introverted mood for your presentation.

You see, in both cases most people would allow themselves to be controlled by the event, rather than deciding to take charge and to be in control of how the event affected them.

Once you attain the state of Laser Visualization, you will be in control of every event in your life, and minor things like a rainy day or a presentation to your boss will not divert you from reaching your goal!

Laser Visualization Changes Everything

Being in a state of Laser Visualization consists basically of imagining things. I use the term *Laser Visualization* because this psychological process can carve new successes and destinies with the most stunning accuracy and efficiency. After you practice the techniques in this chapter, you'll be able to focus your thoughts like a powerful laser beam, drawing into your life whatever you focus on throughout the day.

New research suggests that the superior achievements of famous thinkers may have been more the result of mental conditioning and visualization than of genetic superiority. You can learn to condition your mind in the same way and improve your performance in virtually all aspects of life.

This laser technique enables you to bypass old, outdated inhibitions and access the core realities hidden in your own subconscious. It is believed that the famous physicist Albert Einstein, for example, spent hours *imagining* what it would be like to travel at the speed of light. It was through this technique of visualization that he was able to create his famous theories of time and space.

Nikola Tesla, another great physicist, was said to visualize all of his famous discoveries (such as the principle of the rotating magnetic field) before he made them, and all of his inventions (including wireless communication and fluorescent lights) before he built them.

Much as for these scientific luminaries, visualization can be YOUR inner guide, the internal compass that directs you unerringly toward the important goals of your life. It's already there, waiting in your mind's eye right now, yearning to be developed.

Visualization can make your dream body become a reality

Interestingly enough, we use visualization in our lives every day—sometimes for good purposes, but, more often than not, for uses that stifle our development.

To understand how that happens, let's look first at the Universal Laws of imagination, mind, and achievement. These are the principles that have guided the successes of men and women throughout the ages.

Let me again explain the concept of a Universal Law. A Universal Law is a law that is not refutable by anyone. It cannot be opposed in any way, and it cannot be altered by anyone. We must move in accordance with these laws, just as humans have done since the beginning of time. Perhaps the most visual of these laws to use as an example is the Law of Gravity. When Sir Isaac Newton was sitting under that legendary apple tree and stumbled upon this law, the apple that fell on his head had no choice of direction in which to fall once the twig had snapped. It could not have moved upward or sideways. The Law states that any object that is not significantly affected by air resistance will be drawn directly downward, to the earth. All other Universal Laws are equally unbreakable.

Law Number 1: The mental images and ideas we hold in our minds produce the *physical* reality and the *activities* to which the images correspond.

Law Number 2: A human being always acts in accordance with the mental images and ideas he/she holds and accepts as either true or false, real or imagined, regardless of their source.

"The imagination," according to the great success writer Napoleon Hill, "is literally the workshop wherein are fashioned all plans created by man. The impulse, the desire, is given shape, form and action through the aid of the imagination faculty of the mind."

What Hill is saying is that before we can really achieve something we desire, we must first have an image of that reality already alive in our imagination. And, according to Universal Law Number 1, once the visualization or idea of the thing has been created, willpower will see to it that the *physical* counterpart to the thing is created. You will enable your willpower to create its counterpart in reality: **a dynamically slim, youthful, energetic body.**

We must remember that everything in our world is made up of energy. Your thoughts, for example, are energy. And thought is an energy that can be transferred into its physical equivalent.

A sculptor will have a visualization, an *idea*, of what he or she wants to create before even beginning to shape and mold. A child may dream of being an actress long before she ever takes an acting lesson. Dreams, of course, are forms of visualization. And studies show that people who have a clear idea of what they want are far more likely to achieve it.

We have all seen evidence of this in our own lives. Whenever we have an idea that we think about constantly, our minds cannot help churning out concepts and actions to turn that idea into reality: a better job, a more workable relationship with our spouse or children, a better way of doing something. If we can *imagine* the solution to our problem, we can *create* a solution in reality.

A special note of caution is in order here: The opposite is also true—and must be avoided at all cost! Whenever you consistently think bad thoughts, bad things will be drawn into your life. If you constantly harbor thoughts of your relationship being bad, you will cause your relationship to become bad. If you constantly picture yourself as being fat, out of shape, unhealthy, sickly, or unmotivated, you will draw these things into your life! And this will happen unless you switch from harboring negative thoughts to entertaining positive, successful thoughts.

You can engage in visualization at any time of the day. In fact, when you have become good at this process, you'll be able to hold on to the goals you have visualized, even while you're working, sleeping, talking, driving, etc. And once you become good at this, your mind will actually be stronger and more receptive to your current needs.

Although you could practice visualization at any time, I suggest that you do your visualizing while you're as deeply relaxed as possible, and that you do this as frequently—and for as long a time—as is convenient for you. You don't need to go into a trance-like meditation. What is important is clarity and singularity of focus. In that respect, it's like daydreaming, something we just naturally do all the time. The biggest difference is that daydreaming is a random, almost involuntary preoccupation, whereas Laser Visualization is planned, purposeful, and goal oriented.

The Imagination Can Do Our Bidding

The second principle of visualization is even more important than the first. This law states, in effect, that a person always acts, feels, and performs in accordance with the images in his or her mind, regardless of where they come from. When you think and believe in yourself as a "winner," for example, your mind will retain any thoughts and beliefs that are appropriate to this mindset, and it will automatically discard any thoughts and ideas that are unsupportive.

The second law states, in addition, that the mind *neve*r acts in a vacuum. It will process *any* visualization, any thought or idea it receives, regardless of the source. The subconscious mind makes no distinction whatsoever between constructive and destructive thoughts and images. Nor does it judge whether the material it receives is true or false, real or imagined.

The more important point—and this is a powerfully important discovery—is this: The subconscious will do this with *any* information it gets, **even with images which you purposefully plant in your subconscious**. Using Laser Visualization, you can learn to use your mind to intentionally create whatever you want in your life, including a better, healthier body.

As We Visualize, So We Become

Keep repeating to your son that he is stupid and worthless, and before long he'll reproduce that image in reality. In other words, he'll start behaving as if he *were* stupid and worthless. Since you have been feeding him visualizations of a "loser," he'll start selecting and accepting from his world those images and ideas that support the notion that he is worthless.

On the other hand, tell your son that he is exceptionally bright, and although he may have only average intelligence, he will begin to act on the visualizations you've put into his head and will perform according to this new self-image. He'll actually begin to perform as a better-than-average student.

Again, remember that it makes no difference whether your images are true or false. *If you perceive them* to be true, they will carry full weight with you.

Food for Thought

Feed your mind thoughts about a fat, slovenly body, incapable of serious exercise and metabolic change, and that age-old saying "whatsoever a man sows, that shall he also reap" is sure to be fulfilled. Before you know it, you'll be binging on ice cream and brownies, and continuing your life as a couch potato.

Feed your mind visuals about slimness, health, and a happier, more fit you, and your mind will find harmonizing thoughts, ideas, and actions from the world around it to turn these pictures into the real thing: a permanently thinner you. The winners' circle will soon be yours!

Why not *visualize* yourself as fit, vibrant, and beautiful?

Realizing that your actions, feelings, and behavior are the direct result of the images and beliefs with which you nourish your mind, you have the perfect tool you need to build a better body. By evoking mental pictures of yourself having successfully boosted your metabolism (becoming fit, eating right, and being in good health), you'll provide yourself with the images your willpower needs to turn your goals into reality.

Getting Started

Your first step in controlling your mind–body link through proper visualization is to decide what you want to look like. What do you want to physically and mentally change about yourself? Remember, your body is a direct reflection of the way you see yourself when you close your eyes! Change how you see yourself and you'll change how others see you!

I know what you're thinking: "But I went through this process in an earlier chapter. Why do I have to do it again?" Well, let me make two comments about that:

First, the more you write and re-write your affirmation, your statement of success, and your goals, the more focused you will be and the more honed or polished they will become. If you re-wrote your goals twenty times a day, each day making them crisper and more accurate, you wouldn't be wasting a single second. In fact, you'd be doing more for yourself this way than by almost any other step you could take toward reaching your goals.

Second, what I want you to do in this chapter is different. This exercise will help you take what you've already written and make it clearer and more precise. Remember, the more focused your goals, the faster they will become a reality.

All I want you to do here is to describe in writing the person you have set out to become, in simple, declarative language. And here's the most important thing: write your description of your dream self *as if the changes have already taken place.* Your goal, in the visualization exercises that follow, is to add as many visual and emotional details to this "picture" as possible.

You might write something like this:

> Now that I have lost thirty pounds, my clothes are fitting more loosely. My metabolism is a fat-burning furnace. I'm losing weight, I have tons of energy, and I feel great!

Visualize yourself in such a way that you portray your success as completely and accurately as possible. Picture yourself in happy situations, enjoying your successes as if they were already yours.

Make sure you see this very clearly. You might be able to reinforce your visualization by actually drawing a picture of your goal body.

Finally, believe with all your heart that the object of your visualization, your goal body, is yours—or will become yours. Remember, any disbelief will simply introduce negative energy into the situation and will dilute the power of this exercise. Once you see that you have indeed achieved your ideal body, acknowledge that you made it happen and be proud of yourself!

Now go out and live life in the knowledge that you are already at your goal weight, that you've already achieved your success, and that you're already proud of all you've achieved. Your body will soon resemble the picture that you have in your mind.

How to Visualize

I want you to do just what I've outlined above, and to do it every day for the next thirty days. Set aside a time each day when you can relax, uninterrupted, a time when you can let your imagination run free and wild.

You might choose to do this exercise in the morning before you arise, or perhaps at the end of the day before you go to sleep. For that matter, you can do this exercise at any time of the day. The more positive energy you send out, the more you will get back. That's just the way the Universe works.

Any comfortable spot will do: a bed, a couch, an easy chair, even at your desk. The important thing is that your mind be free from distractions: away from phones, kids, and computers; away from it all.

Find your spot, and then make a conscious effort to relax each part, each muscle of your body, one by one. Start with your head and neck, and work your way down to your toes. This should take several minutes. As you perform this relaxation exercise, take slow, deep breaths. Allow yourself to become as relaxed as possible. Close your eyes and let your thoughts drift inward.

Your First Week

During the first seven days of this exercise, picture as vividly as possible how rewarding and satisfying your life will become when you achieve the body of your dreams. Keep a running list in your personal journal of all the benefits of your maximized metabolism.

Think of how you will behave once you achieve your goal weight, fitness level, or eating regimen. Make these pictures as detailed as possible. Are you confident and self-assured? Are you achieving success in the other areas of your life as well?

See yourself acting confidently and deliberately in those situations that have caused you embarrassment in the past. See yourself behaving with assuredness, poise, and, above all, *determination*, especially in circumstances where you may have previously wilted with trepidation. At the gym. On the track. In a new dress or suit. At a business meeting. At your wedding or high-school reunion.

Hold these pictures in your mind as long as you can. Turn them over again and again. Look for new detail, added dimension, colorful nuance—and, perhaps most of all, rich emotion.

Your Second Week

Emotions are crucial to the process of visualization.

When combined with your emotions, your visualizations will sharpen and intensify your ability to change your ways of thinking and your behavior, much as a magnifying glass focuses and intensifies the rays of the sun.

The need to incorporate your emotions into the process of visualization is precisely the point that most other so-called self-help gurus miss. You see, affirmations in and of themselves don't work, and positive thinking *alone* is practically a waste of your time. As a matter of fact, none of this mental training will do much of anything for you UNLESS you mix emotion in with it! Emotions are the spark plugs that start that beautiful car sitting in your garage. No matter how beautiful that car is, no matter how fast the engine, no matter how many times you wax it, it won't go anywhere without spark plugs. Likewise, your positive self-talk and all your visualization training won't go anywhere in the absence of strong emotions.

I'm thinking about emotions such as love, happiness, confidence, joy, self-respect, etc. When you drench your visualizations with these emotions, they are twice as valuable as goal-directing devices. How do you *feel* when your metabolism is under your complete control? Happy? What emotions do you experience when you show off a sleek, well-toned body? Well, remember the emotions that you experience at times like that. In fact, remember them fifty times a day.

The more you experience those emotions while picturing your goal body, the faster your results will come.

Since Laser Visualization is new to most of you, it will take time and practice to achieve its most important results. Your powers of visualization may have grown diffuse and weak from disuse. But your imagination can become more vivid, more effective, through use and training, just as any muscle or organ of the body becomes stronger through use.

Be particularly careful to focus on visions that reflect your reasons for mastering your metabolism and becoming physically fit, and be sure to add the special leavening agent of *emotion*. Think not just in terms of being thin, but of being *happily and joyously* thin. Or thin and sexy. You know what I mean.

Imagine each benefit in its smallest detail, so that you become thoroughly familiar with every aspect of the idea. By doing so, you will set for yourself a pattern, and create a mold, after which *your inner life will shape your outer life*. You will generate well-beaten mental paths, "habits," along which your visualization can travel in its search for shapely expression. Repeat the same visual pictures again and again, and a new, sexier you will take shape before your very eyes.

Your Third and Fourth Weeks

In the third and fourth weeks, the time you devote to your visualization exercises must grow longer, first to twenty minutes, and then to thirty minutes or more. You see, once you've mastered this technique, you will be holding your image twenty-four hours a day. That twenty- to thirty-minute period of intense training will act simply as a booster, or a refresher, of your actual affirmation or statement of success.

Visualize yourself as being powerfully strong and in control of every aspect of your life. See yourself routinely saying no to junk food and other temptations that slow your metabolism. See how much better you'll look, in full detail—and get emotional about it!

It Works!

Successful users of the program outlined in this book have profited from this technique over and over again. Many were skeptical at first, but in no time at all they found themselves vigorously reducing the gap between their inner and outer selves.

In his book *Psycho-Cybernetics*, Maxwell Maltz recounts the miracles that many men and women have achieved by visualization. His work cites how a salesman increased his sales by 400 percent, simply by *imagining* he was successful; how a world-famous chess player and a professional golfer "practiced" winning plays in their imagination; and how a renowned concert pianist became great by practicing the piano "in his head."

Napoleon Hill, Shakti Gawain, William Atkinson, and Robert Assagioli, as well as many famous students of visualization who came before them, recognized the vital role that visualization plays in achieving lifelong dreams, whether the dream is to develop the perfect body or to make a million dollars.

This daily exercise will lend new determination and resoluteness to your willpower. These visions, rich with desire-supporting emotions, will become new memories, new "tapes" if you will, that your mind will automatically "play" when your program needs a temporary boost. Just as negative "old tapes" can drag you down, these new tapes you create through laser visualization will force your subconscious mind to help you reach your goal.

Before long, you'll see yourself spontaneously acting with confidence and poise. You'll find that you can effortlessly and successfully follow the program and create the new you.

Words of Power

One exercise that is quite helpful in fostering positive visions is called Words of Power. The secret here is to think of the *words* that produce vivid images of success. Only *you* can provide the words, since only *you* know which words have the power to evoke strong, positive mental images of your success—words that are also laden with emotion.

Examples of words of power you might choose are *energetic*, *youthful*, *dynamic*, and *sexy*. You be the judge. To bring these words alive in your imagination, write your words of power in your journal as many times as you can. My guess is that you'll choose two or three words, and that you'll write each of them anywhere from two hundred to four hundred times. Every time you do this, they will be further ingrained in your psyche and the emotions associated with them will be strengthened.

As you begin what appears to be a genuinely tedious task, an interesting thing will happen: your mind will start drifting from the mechanical labor of writing the words, and you'll unconsciously start visualizing what your words of power mean to you.

You'll start daydreaming about how much more sexy and attractive you'll look when you're thin: the clothes you'll wear, the places you'll go, the people you'll meet, and how they'll instantly feel about you. Think about these images and keep writing. They'll keep coming just as long as you keep writing. When the images stop presenting themselves and your mind drifts to another subject, that's the time to move on to the next word.

This is a fabulous exercise. Try it and you'll see! You can even use your words of power while exercising or while eating healthful foods. In fact, just *thinking* about your power words can begin the flow of desire-building images, emotions, and energy.

Selecting Your Power Words

Right now, make up a list of power words, your "dieting vocabulary." Perhaps the words that light up your desire are *skinny*, *trim*, and *attractive*, though you're not limited to selecting words that have something to do with dieting per se. At least some of your power words may be pertinent to successes in other areas of your life that are associated with being very attractive and energized. So be it.

My Personal Words of Power

1. ______________________________

2. ______________________________

3. ______________________________

4. ______________________________

5. ______________________________

Affirmations Spur Your Visualizations

Making daily affirmations is another excellent way to help the visualization process bring about your desired outcome. To affirm something means to state it as the truth. There is always some thought or idea running through your mind that you could affirm. This "self-talk" can be either positive or negative, and it's very often unconscious.

As you're getting dressed in the morning, taking a shower, going about your work, or driving someplace, your mind is thinking thoughts, some of which are positive and some of which are negative. There is no such thing as an "in-between" thought; every thought you have is either a help or a hindrance to achieving your goals. There are no gray areas here.

If you are not in full control, monitoring your thoughts and training yourself to think positively at all times, your mind will take the garbage that others are showering on you and use it to form negative images. The negativity may come from the morning news, or from coworkers, or from any of the persons, places, and events that subconsciously influence you throughout the day. You can put a stop to this influx of negativity by training yourself to think positive thoughts, to feel positive emotions, and to repeat positive affirmations throughout the day—especially the ones that are associated with maximizing your metabolism.

Making affirmations is one way in which we can consciously utilize our self-talk to purposely create good in our lives. They work for the same reason that visualizations work: our subconscious mind has this miraculous ability to translate visualizations into reality, thoughts into results.

An affirmation should be stated in the present, *as if it is already valid*, and it should be repeated as often as possible—many times a day is best. Phrases that begin with "I am" and "I have" are very effective. An affirmation that has to do with good health might go something like this: *I am healthy and well, and every day I feel better and more energized.*

You Can't Go Wrong!

My clients have profited from this technique over and over again. Controlling themselves became easier, and developing the staying power they needed in order to achieve their goals became more natural.

This daily exercise will fan the flames of desire, lending fresh determination and resoluteness to your new diet and exercise regimen. And the visions you experience, rich with desire-supporting emotions, will provide new memories that you can mentally repeat over and over again when you need a mental or physical boost.

Practice Makes Perfect

As you practice these exercises each day, you'll be amazed at how quickly they'll incite your desire to the level that's needed for successful self-change. Moreover, you can do these exercises at any time or in any situation. They'll continue to work for as long as you continue to use them, and they'll point the way to an exciting future—but only if you allow them to do so.

15

Massage Therapy

Let Someone Else Do the Work While You Reap All the Benefits

To many newcomers to the *Maximize Your Metabolism* program, treating yourself to a therapeutic massage may seem to be just a pretentious self-indulgence, the kind of pampering that's to be enjoyed only by those who can afford to frequent a pricey spa or exercise boutique.

The truth is that massage can do a lot of good for anyone, but especially for those who are serious about improving their health, reducing their physical and mental stress, and maximizing their metabolism.

The aim of massage therapy is to work on the body in order to free up the mind, but it also frees up all the toxins stored within your muscles and the destructive stresses that are embedded within your other vital systems. The concept of a mind–body connection dates back to the ancient Chinese, who believed that all illness was the result of imbalance and disharmony between the body and the mind.

German psychoanalyst Wilhelm Reich has probably done as much as anyone to solidify the mind–body link in recent times. Reich, a contemporary of Sigmund Freud, believed that emotions don't just drift through the brain, but that they also show up in the body, often becoming enmeshed in muscles, where they remain unexpressed, thereby creating stress, tension, and mental and physical pain.

To get his patients back in touch with these unexpressed feelings, Reich manipulated and massaged their bodies, putting pressure on certain key areas in an attempt to undo the negative effects that had accumulated. Reich believed that once the toxic deposits due to unexpressed emotional states were broken up and the unpleasant memories of those states were eliminated, he could then proceed to use the more traditional, talk-oriented therapy.

Whatever the origins of massage, it works. It has a tremendous healing effect on both mind and body, and more and more people are turning to massage for relief.

Let's face it, most Americans do things to the extreme. They're so focused on their work that they don't even notice that they've sat all day staring at their computers or performing tedious tasks around the office. Naturally, they end up with taut muscles, a stiff neck, and a backache, and massage works wonders to relieve their pain and tension.

Scientific as well as psychological notions as to why massage is beneficial abound. The most popular theory is that toxins such as lactic acid accumulate in the muscles through normal metabolism and exercise. Most of these toxins are removed by the flow of blood through the body, but knots sometimes form in the muscles, resulting in pain. Stroking, kneading, and other manipulations used in Swedish and other forms of massage bring about the hasty removal of both the knots and the toxins.

Massage Is Catching On

No wonder that in today's go-go, high-stress society, therapeutic massage is rapidly gaining even wider acceptance. The newcomers tend to be people in high-pressure careers, such as middle and upper managers, CEOs, stockbrokers, bond traders, and lawyers. But the list doesn't stop there. Doctors, business owners, housewives, mothers, clerical workers, and people in many other walks of life are availing themselves of massage therapy as a way to increase their productivity while reducing their daily stress. They go to massage therapists because they want to relax and unwind.

Most health clubs and chiropractors' offices have added massage to their menu of treatments. If a prospective client is unable or unwilling to get to one of these types of places for a massage, many of them will bring the massage to the client. In-office and in-home visits are commonplace these days, and they include everything from a full-body massage to just a "chair" massage (a special chair is set up and the client is given a fifteen-minute treatment, without disrobing).

Massage is often combined with modifications to the client's sensory environment. For example, relaxing music, soft colors, and dim lighting can be incorporated into the process. It's all part of a holistic, mind–body approach to good health.

How Massage Helps

Researchers aren't precisely sure about all of the benefits that massage exerts on the human body and mind. But there is no doubt whatsoever that the benefits are significant, or that they are both immediate and long lasting.

By stimulating blood circulation and oxygen flow through the muscles, massage helps to lower blood pressure, speed up healing of injured tissue, and aid in keeping muscles supple. But it is not a panacea, and it is not recommended for those with circulatory ailments. For those of you who are wondering, one thing massage will not do is permanently rub away excess weight.

The list of benefits a given person can expect to attain from one massage session is quite lengthy. The list of benefits one can expect from massage performed on a regular basis is easily twice as long. Those benefits include an increased metabolic rate, which comes about by improving how all of the other bodily systems work.

For example, you've heard the expression "the chain is only as strong as its weakest link." Well, the body can function only as well as *its* weakest link, and the metabolism can be only as healthy as *its* weakest link. Massage helps soothe the stress away from many of our internal organs: the muscles and all of the other systems in our body. When stress is reduced, our body simply functions better.

Here are just a few ways in which it does so:

Massage both calms and relaxes. Part of that has to do with the relaxed environment and the therapeutic context in which the massage generally occurs. This soothing effect is then heightened by the professional yet caring touch of a qualified massage therapist. It works out knots in the muscles, releases physical stress, soothes the mind, and just plain feels good.

Massage promotes flexibility, since many massage routines involve stretching and caressing tired and aching muscle groups. It kneads away stress and improves the elasticity of the muscles.

Massage eases pain, tension, and fatigue for those suffering from a variety of medical conditions, including low-back pain, cancer, and sickle-cell anemia. This pain-reducing capability is thought to be the result, in part, of the ability of massage to increase the body's natural production of the brain chemical serotonin, which is associated with pain reduction.

Massage can relieve respiratory conditions such as asthma and emphysema, according to the Encyclopedia of Natural Healing. It can also balance the nervous system and improve sleep quality.

Circulation and Metabolism

Therapeutic massage is especially beneficial for men and women who want to improve their metabolism, because it improves circulation—and circulation aids proper and effective metabolism. Massage has long been associated with pain reduction; the reason, of course, is that massage alters circulation. Relaxation is a physiological reaction that causes blood vessels to dilate, improving blood flow. In addition, proper massage can increase the flow of oxygen to the skin and muscles, prevent illness by boosting the immune system, and improve the circulation of the lymph and blood vessels, which replenish the tissues with needed nutrients. Blood flow is important to improving the metabolism and oxygenating the blood, as discussed earlier.

Types of Massage

There are literally hundreds of different styles of massage therapy around today, and that number is growing as massage therapists around the world dream up new approaches. There's everything from basic Swedish massage to Rolfing, raindrop massage, and hot-rock therapy. There are probably just as many different types of massage as there are reasons for having a massage performed. What's more, the various massage techniques can be applied either singly or in combination.

Swedish massage, the most familiar technique, uses oils to reduce friction, and it employs long, full strokes along with kneading and pounding motions. In the newly popular Japanese Shiatsu and Chinese acupressure, the fingers are used to apply pressure along certain paths on the body in order to release chi (trapped energy). Other techniques include deep-tissue or structural massage, and reflexology, which focuses on the feet and hands.

For those of you who have no experience with massage therapy, let me say that the therapeutic massage regimen that I recommend involves five basic strokes:

- Effleurage, to smooth and extend muscles
- Petrissage, to knead tense muscles
- Friction, to release knots deep in the muscles
- Vibration, to help minimize tension and fatigue
- Tapotement, to stimulate and excite the muscles

Swedish Massage

Most of us are familiar with the so-called Swedish massage. This is the style we so often see in the movies or on television. It uses long, gliding strokes as well as kneading and friction techniques. Its focus is principally on reducing muscle tension and inducing general relaxation.

Sports Massage

Sports massage, on the other hand, is a newer form of massage therapy that was developed to provide important benefits to those who engage in athletics, whether it be professionals, weekend runners, or weightlifters.

The purpose of sports massage is to help maintain your physical condition; boost your energy, endurance, and metabolism; improve your range of athletic motion; and prevent injuries to your muscles and tendons.

Developed in the 1980s, this industry has grown to such a degree that it's now a major component of sports medicine and a permanent fixture at many professional and amateur sporting events. Visit most exercise and fitness centers today and you'll find therapists who practice sports massage. You'll also encounter them at casual weekend sporting events such as 10K races, not to mention major events such as the Olympic games, Ironman competitions, Goodwill and Pan-American games, bicycle races, and big-city marathons.

Competitive athletes aren't the only ones who can—or should—reap the rewards of sports massage, however. Anyone who exercises on the level that's recommended in this book can benefit from it. In fact, sports massage helps the muscles to deal with the repetitive motions inherent in the aerobic and anaerobic activities that are part of the *Maximize Your Metabolism* program.

Massage, Exercise, and Metabolism

When your muscles are tense, the blood can't flow through them efficiently, so that your body doesn't get the oxygen and nutrients it needs. As a result, your metabolism becomes sluggish, which in turn causes pain, stiffness, spasms, and cramps. Frequent massage can help you perform up to your potential and lower your vulnerability to injury.

Muscles get sore when their fibers become abnormally constricted. This can be due to tension, lack of stretching, or overactivity. Sports massage works to get the kinks out so that muscles can perform optimally.

Deep Muscle Benefits

Sports massage differs from your garden-variety massage in both technique and purpose. A sports massage therapist manipulates the muscles, and the soft tissues around them, to spread out the constricted muscle fibers. This powerful action enhances circulation to those tissues, relaxing the muscles and reducing pain as it promotes the release of endorphins, the body's natural painkillers, into the bloodstream.

As with other types of massage, sports massage improves the flow of lymph fluid, which carries immune-boosting white blood cells and also filters out toxins and waste products. Active people especially need their systems cleared of waste products such as lactic acid.

Lactic acid is one of the by-products of physical activity. It's the end product in the metabolism of glucose during the anaerobic production of energy. Muscles give off lactic acid during exercise; as a result, it can build up in the body. Eventually, the body will rid itself of such by-products on its own. In fact, as your body adapts to increased levels of exercise, it also improves in its ability to remove lactic acid from the system. In the meantime, massage speeds up that process, and so the muscles are more quickly prepared for the next bout of activity.

Sports-massage therapists use a particular combination of massage strokes, timing them in a certain way in order to heal and relax the muscles while energizing the body. Different techniques are employed, depending on whether the massage is being given before an exercise session or just for purposes of relaxation.

When to Have a Massage

Whenever you feel tense, achy, or out of sorts, a massage can do you wonders. Massage can also become a regular part of your metabolic-enhancing routine if you incorporate it into your weekly or bimonthly regimen.

Getting the Right Touch

Any massage that you receive will be no better than the skill and technique of the person who delivers it. Here's what you should look for in booking your massage:

First, check with your local department of health about the regulation of massage in your area, and find out what types of credentials a massage therapist needs in order to practice. In some localities, massage therapists need to be licensed by the state, while other areas rely on licensing by the county or city, and still others require nothing!

Second, determine whether your prospective massage therapist has the proper licensure and certification. Professionals should be certified in either "therapeutic massage" or "body work" by the independent National Certification Board for Massage. Make sure your chosen massage therapist has completed at least a two-year academic program in the art of massage and has had at least the minimum number of hours of practical training required to become a Registered Massage Therapist (RMT).

If you want a proper sports massage, it may be a good idea to insist that your therapist be a member of the American Massage Therapy Association (AMTA). To check on practitioners in your area, you can visit the AMTA on the Web, at www.amtamassage.org.

Third, seek the recommendations of others. If you're scouting around for a therapist, there is nothing that beats references from friends. Word-of-mouth advertising nearly always proves to be beneficial when it comes to selecting someone who will be laying their hands on you. Knowing that your massage therapist has delivered superior services to others helps ensure that he or she will deliver the same to you.

Although the list of massage therapies given above is incomplete, it does form a basis for you to get started in your search for a technique that fits both your lifestyle and your personality.

My suggestion at this point is to do a bit of research into massage therapists in your area. Try to choose someone who is within reasonable distance of your home or place of work, and be sure that both the therapist and his/her studio fit your needs. Then relax, and let the therapist do the work for you. By the end of just one visit, you should be able to tell whether you've chosen well—and you will probably have made a good friend, someone who can work with you to *Maximize your Metabolism.*

16

Getting Yourself to Exercise Regularly

Failure to Exercise Is Not an Option

Failure is not an option when a parent
is teaching a child to walk.
Let's make a commitment to each other:
failure is not an option when we're striving to
reach our health and fitness goals either.

This book seeks to demonstrate that exercise bestows a myriad of benefits upon the exerciser, beginning with a more controllable and user-friendly metabolic rate and extending to a full range of outcomes that have personal excellence as their aim. Men and women who engage in regular exercise tend to enjoy better health and longevity, extraordinary freedom from disease and debility, and enhanced psychological well-being, all of which help form the cornerstone of their other achievements in life.

Millions of Americans take these benefits to heart. More than a hundred million Americans are swimmers, seventy-five million are bicyclists, seventy-five million work out at health clubs, and thirty-five million are joggers. One survey shows that a whopping 40 percent of all Americans claim to exercise regularly.

It has been my experience, after years of working with people, that some tend to lose themselves in their workout, while others seem to find themselves.

This is why it seems surprising that exercise is not part of the daily routine for most of the people who participate in health and fitness surveys. Such studies indicate that the majority of people are woefully inactive. For example, only 22 percent of Americans are active at a level that's recommended for good health. Many folks exercise at a level of exertion that ebbs and flows with the intensity of their desire to lose weight. The majority of adults in our great country who are over the age of twenty-five are almost completely sedentary.

Interestingly enough, most people believe in the value of exercise and what it can do for them, both physically and psychologically. Even many of the holdouts who don't exercise think they'd be more attractive and self-assured if they did. The majority of those who engage in exercise on a regular basis report significant benefits in terms of enhanced energy, mood, and creativity; improved health and body shape; greater control of stress; and even a more active social life.

How We Begin and How We Fade

Most people typically begin their exercise programs in response to nagging problems caused by weight gain. For many of us, New Year's Day is the starting date for a flurry of activity in this regard, as we become penitent over too much holiday eating and entertaining—and long stretches of winter idleness—and plunge headlong into exercise programs. Health clubs and gyms experience a resurgence of membership, while jogging and walking paths become crowded with would-be fitness enthusiasts. Manufacturers of exercise equipment and purveyors of weight-loss programs vie elbow to elbow for the available advertising time on radio and television and in print media. For many folks, however, the motivation to exercise fades within a few short weeks.

Why We Fade

Perhaps the most common reason given by sedentary people for avoiding exercise is a lack of time. Many studies have been conducted in which people who drop out of fitness programs blame time constraints. A nationwide Gallup Poll conducted in 1989 revealed that 39 percent of respondents said their reason for not exercising was that they "had no time for such activity." Twenty percent of the respondents felt that they got enough exercise in their daily routine, hence that they had no need to do anything extra. Another study, undertaken by Melpolmene Institute, a women's fitness and health organization, reached a similar conclusion: time was perceived to be a major limiting factor.

Is it true that the vast majority of people in this country don't have time to fit an exercise period into their day on a regular basis? I don't believe so, and neither do many other experts.

One of the foremost researchers on the phenomenon of the failure to stick with an exercise program is Dr. Roy Shephard of the University of Toronto. In two separate studies, Dr. Shephard points out that although people *say* that lack of time is their major obstacle to exercising, it's really just an excuse. The average American, says Dr. Shephard, has between fifteen and eighteen hours of leisure time per week, and often has the TV on for *seven hours a day* at home.

By strictly adhering to and implementing the practices laid out in this manual, not only will you gain the motivation you need to get fired up about your fitness-filled future, but you will also experience major changes in your body that will keep that fire lit for years to come.

What Experience Has Proved

Throughout the years that I've been in the exercise and fitness business, I've seen literally thousands of men and women start and sustain meaningful, long-term exercise programs. I've also seen my share of dropouts. My overall conclusion is that if you can sustain your exercise program for a good, solid thirty to sixty days, you have an excellent chance of making it a permanent part of your lifestyle, and of seeing dramatic results if it is done properly. Here are some tips for making the process a little easier:

Find an activity you enjoy. This seems so obvious to me, and yet millions of would-be exercisers base their choice of exercise regimen on all the wrong criteria. Instead of finding exercises they consider to be enjoyable, they choose them solely according to the number of calories they'll burn up, or how trendy looking the gym or health club appears. Then, when the novelty wears off, so does the commitment.

Many research studies have shown that if people pursue an activity they don't like, they won't stick with it for long at a time—and they'll eventually abandon it altogether. To avoid this kind of exercise burnout, start with exercises that you truly enjoy. Whether it's running, walking, or using exercise equipment such as free weights, make sure you like what you're doing and that it provides the results you're looking for.

Make exercising convenient. Virtually everyone has a busy lifestyle. In fact, just about everyone would say that their day is completely filled. In order to add an exercise program, you may have to eliminate a less important activity (such as watching TV). If your day is too crowded, you'll soon be looking for excuses to skip your exercise program. At first, that might mean skipping just an exercise session or two. Later, however, you're likely to let entire weeks go by without exercising. Finally, you'll go back to the old sedentary lifestyle that you promised you'd give up.

Don't let that happen to you. The more convenient you can make your exercise routine, the better. That means scheduling your exercises at a *time of day* when you'll consistently do them and on *days of the week* when you can exercise regularly.

Set goals and chart your progress. "Nothing succeeds like success," said French novelist Alexandre Dumas. The more success we achieve in any endeavor, the more likely we are to continue with it. This notion is extremely important, especially when it comes to exercising our bodies and building up our metabolism.

Goals are the mental roadmap that your mind uses to attain its desired ends. Goals are the conduits that funnel all of your physical and mental energies toward a single purpose.

A wealth of professional research has demonstrated that being precise about health and fitness goals improves the chances of sticking to an exercise program. Perhaps the best way to do this is to use a journal or logbook to chart your progress. Making frequent (daily, if possible) entries in your journal will help keep your motivation high and prevent your commitment from waning.

Do imagination exercises. This is another useful way to enhance your motivation. You may already be familiar with this psychological technique from some weight-loss class you have attended. The method is simple and easy to follow. We've spoken about this earlier, but because of its importance I'll briefly touch upon it here.

First, find a quiet place where you can relax without being interrupted, preferably in a comfortable chair in a private room. Then close your eyes and *imagine* yourself with the body that you desire (and that will soon be yours!): the clean, sculpted look, with well-defined muscles that are lean, flexible, and ready for any kind of movement you might choose. Visualize how you'll look with no excess body fat, and see yourself in your new body, engaging in your favorite activities to your heart's desire. Imagine how your family, friends, and coworkers will treat the "new you." Hear them congratulating you, and get a sense of how that feels. In short, get excited!

Try to make your visualizations as *specific* as possible, and try to drench your images with lots of *emotion*. How do you *feel* when people compliment you on your new, slimmer look? What emotions race through your whole being when your increased stamina and productivity enable you to do all those wonderful things you've been yearning to do?

Perform this exercise several times a day. You may be capable of doing it in as little as one minute, but you should work your way up to thirty minutes each time. You'll be surprised at how well it will enhance your ability to stick to your exercise plans and almost magically bring about the results you desire.

Take responsibility. Sticking to your exercise program is nobody's responsibility but your own. Nobody can do it for you, and no one else is to blame if you miss a workout. That means you've got to take responsibility for each and every workout, as well as for the results. You've got to become proactive in your approach, planning in advance in order to ward off problems and temptations that might beset you. Then one to three months hence, when you find that people are complimenting you and noticing you from across the room, you'll have the immense satisfaction of knowing that your accomplishments were of your own doing, not someone else's. You're the one to whom people will give all the credit when you succeed. By the same token, you're the one they'll hold responsible for your failure if you don't stick to your exercise regimen or you start skipping workouts.

In the end, what it all boils down to is this: If you have to actually tell people that you work out, your workout is not working well enough. But if people begin complimenting you and asking about how you work out or what type of diet you're on, then you'll know that all your efforts have been worthwhile.

My goal so far in this book has been to give you all the techniques that truly work and cut out the ones that are just plain worthless. The only proof I have that these techniques work are the piles of compliments that are heaped on my clients by friends and family. Just think: if you stick with the *Maximize Your Metabolism* program, you'll be the next person to receive all those delicious compliments.

One thing you need to plan for is what you will do when that report simply "must be done" by tomorrow morning and your regular time to exercise is at 5:30 P.M. today. And what will you do to pump yourself up when your interest dwindles?

One excellent suggestion is that you enlist a friend to exercise with you. Going it alone may be perfectly fine for the person who's into long-distance running, but partnering with someone may be a far better solution for those who follow the *Maximize Your Metabolism* program. If you don't have a workout partner, then by all means use your fictitious mentoring group.

In the past, I've forced some of my clients to switch gym bags (contents included!) with their exercise partner. That way, neither of them can exercise unless the other shows up. Remember: *plan in advance*. Then when problems crop up, you'll have ready-made solutions at your disposal, thus staving off the possibility of a missed workout.

Let others help you. One of the easiest ways to stick to your program of exercising to maximize your metabolism is to draw upon the motivational reservoir found in *others*; you don't absolutely have to go it alone.

In this respect, employers have an important role to play. Studies show that jobs and careers are placing increased pressures on employees. As a result, lack of time is seen as a major constraint to regular exercise.

Many employers are solving this problem—and ending up with employees who are more productive—by offering one or more exercise or fitness options at company expense. Among such offerings are installation of a company-owned fitness center, giving employees time off for exercise, and paying for all or a portion of a health-club membership. Check with your employer to see what is presently offered, or what could be offered in the future if employee interest is sufficient.

The support of family and friends has also been identified as being quite influential in encouraging relatively inactive people to become more active. Perhaps the single most effective form of encouragement is the presence and companionship of a friend or relative at the times when you engage in exercise or other physical activity. Many people find that their spouse is the one who provides the greatest support in this regard.

Keep it fun. This is probably the best advice of all! I realize that the techniques outlined in this book are not easy, but they work nonetheless, and they work better than any other combination of techniques I've come across. If you need to find ways to keep your routine fun in order to stick to it, then challenge yourself to do just that. By reading this book and studying what it has to offer, you've already surmounted the biggest hurdle and you've created the cornerstone for a powerful health and fitness regimen. Now all you have to do is *keep it fun*.

One way you can do that is by varying the music you listen to while working out. Put yourself in charge of the tunes you hear, by using a portable CD player while you exercise. Or you could join two different health clubs and then alternate between them, spending a week at each one. You be the judge, and, as the saying goes, "Just do it!"

My health club provides free subscriptions to several motivational e-mail newsletters (some daily, some weekly) to help the members stick to their programs. As a reader of this book, you too are invited and encouraged to sign up for one or more of these newsletters today—they're free, and they're well worth it.

17

Take Action: Your Motivational Challenge

Become Your Perfect Self—Starting Today!

"The difference between a successful person and others is not a lack of strength, but rather in a lack of will."

—Vince Lombardi

In this book I have placed a great deal of emphasis on the role that both diet and exercise play in permanently maximizing your metabolism. Now I want to go one step further. In order for you to accomplish any goal, you must keep pushing, every single day. In this program, as in life in general, motivation is key.

One of the truly legendary motivators of our time was the great coach of the Green Bay Packers, Vince Lombardi. In his long and illustrious career, Vince never put forth anything but his best effort. Moreover, he expected the same of his players and staff. In one of his many motivational speeches, he said:

> Winning is not a sometime thing; it's an all-the-time thing. You don't win once in a while; you don't do things right once in a while; you do them right all the time. Winning is a habit. Unfortunately, so is losing.

Lombardi then went on to say:

> There is no room for second place. There is only one place in my game, and that's first place. The object is to win—to beat the other guy. . . . I believe in God, and I believe in human decency. But I firmly believe that any man's finest hour, the greatest fulfillment of all that he holds dear, is that moment when he has worked his heart out in a good cause and lies exhausted on the field of battle—Victorious.

Motivating Yourself to Victory

I want you to be victorious in this program. Just how close at hand that victory *is*—in this or any other program you'll try, and no matter what aspect of your life it pertains to—hinges on the effort you're willing to put in to achieve it. If you harness the awesome power of your motivation, you can and will achieve anything you want in life.

Fortunately, the techniques outlined in this book will go a long way in providing much of the motivation you'll need. What I have observed in my many years in the health and fitness field is that men and women who begin to take care of their lives tend to do so in ever-widening spheres. They start small, and, compelled by their successes, they become interested in, motivated for, and more capable of other forms of self-improvement. Their motivation, when properly harnessed and trained, becomes a self-perpetuating phenomenon.

I have personally witnessed many clients who, having taken up strength training, group exercise classes, hiking, or swimming as an adjunct to their metabolic rejuvenation, continued in these activities long after attaining the metabolic rate they were aiming for.

The crucial point is this: Not all Americans who have committed themselves to a lifestyle that includes regular exercise are pursuing exercise for its own sake, nor are they necessarily undertaking their exercise program in a quest for the shapeliest body in the locker room or the shortest time on the marathon course. On the contrary, I've found that many people who exercise do so because exercise transforms their lives and helps them become the *best human beings they can be*.

How does this happen? Exercise provides a vital link to improving both our body and our mind. *Exercising makes us feel good about ourselves.* And when we *feel* good about ourselves, we perform better in every other area of our lives. In fact, we become

- More ambitious
- More creative
- More confident
- More energetic
- Better able to cope with life's adversities

- More likely to be honest with ourselves—and honest and fair in our dealings with everyone around us

And, of course, there are so many other attributes that could be included in this list.

The Pursuit of Excellence

Though I wrote this book as both a motivational mainspring and a manual of the most up-to-date methods for generating massive improvements in metabolism, each and every one of my clients has gone on to apply the material contained herein to the improvement of other aspects of their life. I suggest that you do the same. Look upon the program outlined in this book as your opportunity to accept responsibility for your fate and to set out to achieve a state of well-being that comes from a balance of winning in *all* departments of your life: your career, your family, your friendships, your health, and your appearance. It all begins with your ability to master your metabolism.

The reality is that all of us can take charge of our lives and our destinies through a planned program of building our self-motivation. But make no mistake about it: self-motivation is not easy, and it is *not what gets you results*, but it *is* the essential spark that ignites the flame. There can be no blazing fire without a spark, and there can be no accomplishment without motivation. And the stronger the motivation, the greater the accomplishment!

Tips for Motivational Success

The point of this chapter is to refresh your memory about some of the important motivational techniques we talked about in earlier chapters. Your challenge is to put them to good use in your life, starting right now (that is, if you haven't already made them a part of your everyday life).

Affirmations

Throughout this entire book, I've tried to include important steps to help you reprogram your thinking, envision yourself as you would like to look, and then actually affirm your "picture" of yourself. Brian Tracy, one of the world's leading experts on personal success, has said:

> Affirmations are hard to do because people have a natural tendency to return to homeostasis, to what is comfortable, to

> avoid change. But habits are learned and can be unlearned. If you put in three weeks repeating [affirmations] to yourself, you'll be amazed at the results. The formula for affirmations is to put what you want to happen in the first person, present tense, in a positive statement, as if it has already taken place. "I weigh 165 pounds." "I am earning $40,000." "I am a non-smoker."

Don't fall into the trap Tracy talks about. Don't take the easy way out. Break new ground in your life. Use the power of affirmation to keep yourself focused and motivated.

Goal Statements

Another powerful strategy you can use to build motivation is the formulation of a goal statement. In my opinion, goal statements form the heart of the famous *Think and Grow Rich* program created by Napoleon Hill. In case you're not aware of who Napoleon Hill was, he was born into poverty in 1883, in a one-room cabin in rural Virginia. When he was only ten years old, his mother died. Two years later, his father remarried. He began his writing career at age thirteen as a "mountain reporter" for small-town newspapers and went on to become one of America's most beloved motivational authors. Faced with enormous disadvantages and pressures himself, he dedicated more than twenty-five years of his life to pinning down the reasons why so many people fail to achieve true financial success and happiness in their life. Of course, he became fabulously wealthy in the process.

Hill advised his readers to *write down* their goals and read them aloud every day, just as I have advised you to do. His approach was new to his era. Since that time, of course, millions of people have used similar techniques to help themselves achieve success—in every area of life—just as you are now using such techniques to help you achieve all of your health and fitness goals. You should be proud of yourself; you're in good company.

Brian Tracy offers similar advice:

> Just like working out, you can build up your mental muscles by exercising them. Take 3 × 5 index cards and write down your goals. As incredible as it seems, this creates a force field around you that draws in people and circumstances that help. That sounds mystical, but think about the most powerful forces in the universe that are invisible, mysterious, and yet real, like love or gravity. To skeptics, I say, "Try out these

things for thirty days, and simply draw pragmatic conclusions." My ideas are based on what happens, not theory. I'm telling you what successful people really do.

Spending Time with Winners

Another point I have emphasized, and which I'll underscore here, is to get busy spending time with "winners": in person, in books, on the Net, wherever. Listen to what Anthony Robbins, a famous motivational speaker, said about this concept at one of his seminars:

> Whom you spend time with is who you become. If you hang out with firecrackers who see every setback as a challenge and an opportunity to try something better, you'll become a firecracker who sees every setback as a challenge and an opportunity to try something better. If you hang out with schleps who sit around all day kvetching about their problems and who see every setback as proof they are once more getting fiddled by the fickle finger of fate, then you'll become a schlep.

Robbins reiterates some other tips we've emphasized in this book:

> Events in your life don't count as much as the decisions you make about them. Don't be a victim. Take responsibility for everything that happens in your life.
>
> Focus is reality. Whatever you focus on, you feel. The point is that the mind doesn't know the difference between something you vividly imagined and something you actually experienced. So, if you vividly imagine yourself succeeding, your mind is conned into believing that you have already succeeded.

If you do as Robbins prescribes, success will soon follow.

Laser Visualization and Modeling

More than fifty years ago, plastic surgeon Dr. Maxwell Maltz had a revelation after witnessing behavioral and personality changes in his patients who had been involved in disfiguring accidents or had undergone corrective surgery: how you see and what you believe about your self-image controls absolutely what you can and cannot accomplish.

As you learned in the chapter on visualization, visualizing yourself in your mind's eye is a crucial first step in turning your goal body into reality. Maltz takes this a step further. He says the habits and actions you associate with your self-image cannot be changed or overcome without conscious effort, positive thinking, and willpower:

> The person who has a "fat" self-image—whose self-image claims to have a "sweet tooth," to be unable to resist "junk food," who cannot find the time to exercise—will be unable to lose weight and keep it off no matter what he tries to do consciously in opposition to that self-image.

What you must do in order to win is to "reset" the facts about your self-image, from those that portend failure to those that exude success. Modeling your behavior after that of successful people also has the effect of implanting new, more motivational "pictures" in your mind. According to Maltz, this is like the intended action of a heat-seeking missile: you aim and launch it, and it effectively hits its goal.

The powerful strategies I've outlined in this book need a formula to make them work. Here it is:

"I am responsible."

Until you fully believe that nothing occurs by accident, and that you must accept responsibility for every event in your life every day, you will be virtually incapable of performing at a level that's anywhere near your true potential. Once you understand this fact, however, everything will be clearer and your goals will seem to rush toward you.

Your success in fitness, health, and every other area of your life begins in your mind, the most powerful instrument of change on this planet. So powerful in fact, that it has abilities and powers that you're not even aware of. You were born with these powers, but you may never have learned how to master them.

Self-motivation is a matter of choice. Moreover, it's a personal responsibility that you must shoulder. That is, making the right kinds of changes in your life is *your responsibility*. Nobody can do it for you, and you certainly owe it to yourself to make it happen.

Successful living is available to all those who are willing to disregard the negative feelings that tend to hold them back. The energy to reach our goals is generated by closing our mind to all negative "self-talk" and flooding it with our personal success statement.

Successful motivation is not a born-again experience. Rather, it is something that develops from refusing to cave in to negative impulses. It means taking positive action, and doing the right things over and over again until success is yours.

Top motivational speakers such as Zig Ziglar agree. In his book *Success For Dummies,* Ziglar says that by creating goals and developing the right mental attitudes through positive visualization, we can achieve success in *any* environment.

The biggest obstacle to success is feeling that you're not good enough, or comparing yourself unfavorably to others. The psychologist Abraham Maslow said that the story of the human race is one of people selling themselves short. Don't make that mistake!

Your Future Is What You Make of It

To build and sustain motivation, you must have a structured program of activities that reinforce your efforts to take control of your life. Leaving elements of this program to chance is, without question, the worst thing you can do. Anything left to chance will soon be forgotten in the crush of daily events. Use this book as your guide. Use the structure that has now been integrated into your life (through the various types of activities you've encountered in the *Maximize Your Metabolism* program, such as goal setting, journaling, visualizing, dieting, exercising, etc.) to guide your future decisions.

Keep in mind, however, that this book was not designed to be read like a military field manual, nor were the various activities presented in the book intended to be treated as a precise set of instructions to be followed to the letter. This book actually gives you only an *outline*, which then has to be personalized according to your particular goals and circumstances.

And remember this: Even though building motivation is a long-term pursuit, you need only make about thirty consecutive days' worth of consistent efforts in order to ingrain the skill of successful self-motivation into your life. Practice these principles for the next month, and chances are that you'll develop a lifetime of successful motivation in the process.

The Decision Is Now Yours

The decision to incorporate this challenge—and keep on using it—is now yours to make. You can keep sliding along, groping and coping with mediocre performance and less-than-satisfactory results. Or you can step out, away from the crowd, and start charting your own successful destiny.

You can do it. I know you can. Don't wait for someone else to set you free. You have the power within you to make your dreams come true.

George Bernard Shaw made the following astute observation:

> People are always blaming circumstances for what they are. I don't believe in circumstances. The people who get what they want in this life are the people who get up and look for the circumstances they want. And if they can't find them, they make them.

I've been teaching the kinds of techniques that are found in this book for over fifteen years, and in the last couple of years I've provided information—in the form of manuals and books like this one—to hundreds of my clients around the United States. I'm very pleased and grateful for all the thank-you letters I've received from clients who have achieved astonishing results.

I know literally hundreds of people who have made great strides in their health and fitness results with the information you now hold in your hands. However, I also have to tell you that there are failures: people who habitually buy books and tapes, join one health or weight-loss club after another, or try everything from subliminal suggestion to neuro-linguistic programming but never put a single foot forward to take action.

Why is it that some people succeed with this information while others in virtually the same situation fail? Actually, that question has triggered the growth of a whole industry: the motivational industry. Icons in this industry have studied this phenomenon for centuries. The most widely recognized leaders in the field include Brian Tracy, Jim Rohn, Mark Victor Hansen, Earl Nightingale, Anthony Robbins, Dr. Tony Alessandra, Napoleon Hill, Dr. Deepak Chopra, Stephen Covey, Les Brown, Bob Proctor, and Dr. Dennis Waitley—just to name a few.

A friend of mine, Michael Monroe Kiefer, wrote a book entitled *The Powermind System* in which he lists four Essential Personality Traits for High Achievement. He states that anyone who sets out to become a high achiever, in any area of life, can succeed only by focusing on **personal responsibility, personal honor, self-discipline, and persistence**.

The difference between a person who has just skimmed this book and someone like you who has made it all the way through from beginning to end (and, I hope, doing each of the exercises and making the sorts of changes in your life that we spoke of along the way) is that the person who has just scratched the surface is lacking in one or more of these four personality traits.

You must take full responsibility for everything that happens to you in life, including your weight, your looks, and your metabolism. This may seem shallow. I realize that there are horrible things happening in this world. I know that world peace is threatened by one bellicose group after another. I am aware of the fact that hunger and disease are widespread. I know how hard it can be to handle the stresses that crop up in the workplace. And I realize that it may seem trivial—perhaps even selfish—to pay so much attention to your appearance and your personal health to the almost total exclusion of all these important issues.

Well, let me tell you something: Your appearance, health, fitness level, and mental awareness are what enable you to be successful in life. And the more success you have, the more people you can help and the more you can control your destiny.

People who consistently fail at reaching their health and fitness goals usually refer to success as a matter of luck, fate, or coincidence. Or they claim that others have some advantage over them. You, on the other hand, are one of those rare individuals who are keenly aware of the fact that success is definitely not an accident.

In writing this book, I set out to create a cadre of **in**dependents, not to breed a following of **de**pendents. This book is all about taking control and personal responsibility, and it has supplied you with all the tools you need to achieve success in every area of your life, starting with your health. You are now in control of your life and your metabolism, because you have assumed responsibility for reaching your goals.

When I say that you have *all* the tools you need, I mean it. I have held nothing back (fortunately, I didn't *need* to hold anything back) for inclusion in a sequel to this book. Everything I wanted to impart to you is right here, between the front and back covers of this one little volume. There will no further books forthcoming until (and unless) I make new discoveries that will further help you to reach your health and fitness goals. Moreover, any new discoveries that I make and/or new techniques that I develop will be posted on my Web site. (Another way to get that information is to contact me directly, at my office.)

The demand for my services far exceeds my time and energy, so I get to hand pick the people whom I choose to work with, the ones I see as having a true desire to follow a proven system in its entirety. That ability to be selective is what gave me the freedom to produce this book. You see, my reason for writing it was not to create a demand for my services but rather to equip you with the tools necessary for you to succeed on your own—for you to be *in control of your metabolism.*

I really hope you'll pick up the ball and run with it. I look forward to hearing of your successes—and possibly even meeting you someday. In fact, I would like for us to have a continuing relationship, so I urge you to subscribe to one of my newsletters, which are my conduit for maintaining a continuing health and fitness dialogue with my clients and the reading public.

For those of you who have made it this far in the program, please visit me online (at www.MaximizeYourMetabolism.com) to **obtain further information about my newsletters and to receive a special gift I have reserved just for you**. This Web site was developed for the express purpose of sharing ground-breaking knowledge with you—and so that I could extend to you my very best offers on other books and tapes that I think you may find useful.

Thank you for investing in this book, and thank you for reading and learning from it. Now move on to the final chapter, the one that incorporates all that we've discussed so far: the one that's entitled "Seven Days to Shape Your Life and Your Body."

18

Seven Days to Shape Your Life and Your Body

Multiply Your Metabolic Rate Every Day for the Next Seven Days!

Seven days to build your metabolism,
develop high levels of energy,
overcome every past dieting barrier, eliminate stress,
unlock your true potential, and so much more . . . .
This chapter puts it all together and lays it out
in an easy-to-follow format.

At last, you have all the pieces of the metabolic puzzle. Put them together and you've got a powerful blueprint to boost your metabolism to sizzling levels and elevate your health, fitness, and general well-being to an all-time high.

Still, *reading* this material will do nothing unless you *put it to work* in your life. That's why I've created this important chapter. It will help you crystallize your thinking about what I've tried to teach you throughout this book, and then to immediately apply that knowledge in your everyday life. Finally, it will give you specific exercises that will instantly put you on the path to success.

Each day is a new day, and each day you have the same basic choices. The way you handle those choices will determine whether or not you are successful. If you follow the rules and guidelines in this chapter, you will develop a certain "momentum of success," and without a doubt you will achieve your health and fitness goals.

In this chapter, I've laid out activities or exercises for you to do. Each day that you successfully follow the outline presented here, you'll be drawn closer to your goal.

One note of caution: don't move on to the next day's program until you've completed the current day's activities. Even more importantly, complete the current day's activities in full *on the current day*; don't postpone any of them. Make the commitment to become a person of action, starting right now!

In all my years of training and developing people, I've found that the majority of failures happen at this point. You might think that's a depressing—almost demotivating—way to start this chapter, but let's look at it another way: Everyone is driven by both pain and pleasure. My job right now is to show you both. The pain is that this is the point where most failures occur; the pleasure, on the other hand, is that this is the point where all successful people excel and run to the finish line. This is where it all happens. And it's not only quite exciting but also pretty damned motivating if you're truly dedicated!

Maximize Your Emotions

Not a moment goes by in life without emotions, and those emotions have specific effects on our health. Today, day one, we'll take control of our health by taking control of our emotions.

Day One. In the first day of our weeklong goal-setting/action-taking program, I want you to focus entirely on your emotional health. All you'll have to do is study the emotions that you normally experience, and then focus on wiping out the negative ones and boosting the positive ones.

You can help this process along by repeating an affirmation such as the following:

> I am so happy weighing _____ pounds. I eat only healthful foods and drink lots of plain, fresh water. People comment about how great I look, and that makes me feel energized.

Emotions, you'll recall, are the key to our hormonal responses, so when you repeat your affirmation, be sure to get excited about it. When we're depressed, our hormones, glands, and related systems unite to keep us in a depressed state. On the other hand, a heightened enthusiasm for life does just the opposite, and that's why it's absolutely essential to the process of raising our metabolism.

A big part of achieving metabolic success is that of managing your own emotions. You can take active steps to turn all of your feelings into assets that will enhance your health, especially your metabolism. One of the best-kept secrets as to how you can master your emotions is the use of visualization. The more clearly you can visualize yourself acting out and looking like that "person" you describe in your affirmations, the more excited you'll become.

Whenever you repeat your affirmations, make a point of actually seeing yourself happy, weighing your goal weight and dressed in clothing that you think will flatter your physique. Most importantly, be sure to visualize other people remarking on how great you look and congratulating you on your new body, and then experience how good that feels.

Here's an extremely important point:

You are in charge of every emotion you have this day (and night).

We humans all have equal access to everything the universe has to offer, and the resources we've been given in order to deal with people and events in our everyday life are about the same. We all have exactly the same amount of time in each day, more or less the same obstacles to face each day, and practically the same set of mental capabilities for overcoming those obstacles and helping us make good use of our time.

What makes a person great is how much control they exert over their emotions. In other words, no one can control your emotions but you. If someone cuts you off on the highway, how do you react? You're in control of your reaction, and that reaction causes a whole chain of events to take place within your body that will have a significant effect on the functioning of your metabolism. If you curse and get mad, then your body will internalize this emotion and react accordingly. If you simply make adjustments in your driving, become more aware of your surroundings, and refrain from getting angry, then your metabolism, hormones, glands, and all the other systems in your body will have a greater capacity to function at peak level.

The upshot of all this is that getting our metabolism to function at its best is a direct result of how well we control our emotions.

I'll guarantee you that the healthiest people in the world realize this fact, and, regardless of whether they think about it actively or simply have it tucked away in their subconscious mind, they are living in a harmonious way and are in control of how they react to situations. They never allow a situation or another person to dictate their responses to the particular hand of cards that life deals out to them on any given day.

Our three-pronged approach

You may recall that in the chapter on emotions it was noted that emotional management can be made easier by a simple, three-pronged approach: a program of physical fitness, effective time management, and self-image development. And keep in mind that it's rather difficult to maintain a negative *emotion* when your *actions* are positive. In fact, what I consider to be one of today's greatest discoveries is the fact that the human mind cannot entertain a negative thought at the same time that it's focused on a thought that's positive. The two just cannot coexist. It's up to you to choose what thoughts you will allow yourself to focus on, each and every minute of each and every day.

Today's assignment

1. Keep a journal with you all day long. In it, list every type of emotional experience you have. Next to each emotion you list, keep track of how long that emotion lasts and how many times you experience it in the course of the day.
2. Answer the following questions in your journal: What does your perfect body look like? How does it feel to be in the best shape you've ever been in (in your entire life)?
3. List what you will give up in return for achieving your goals.
4. What is your goal date, the date on which you intend to have achieved your ideal body?
5. Prepare, in writing, a detailed and carefully designed plan of action for achieving the body that you envision for yourself. Be sure your plan of action is both specific and achievable.
6. In a single paragraph, summarize the answers to all the questions given above. Make sure your summary is positive and expressed in the present tense. Get excited as you write it out. Remember: by following what I say, you will achieve the results you're aiming for.

7. Read your summary out loud ten or more times in an excited, passionate, obsessive state of mind.

Your mind is the key to all your emotions and the key to achieving all your goals. Keeping your mind in a positive state is vital to achieving anything worthwhile in life.

It's Time to Go on a Cleanse

Nothing that's great can be built on a weak foundation. Building a strong health and fitness foundation starts with first cleaning out your digestive system.

Day Two. In the chapter on cleansing, I began the process of renovating your metabolic system by describing how you should thoroughly cleanse your digestive tract.

Everyone needs to move their bowels at least twice a day, but your goal is to have as many bowel movements as the number of meals you eat in a day's time. If you eat three meals a day, you should have three bowel movements a day. Eating six times per day (large or small meals) means six movements per day.

I realize that having that many bowel movements is far from the norm in our society and may seem rather strange or unusual, but not if you consider what the typical American lifestyle consists of: eating fast food, getting all stressed out, sleeping poorly, and getting little or no exercise. Thankfully, neither you nor I—nor anyone else who follows the program presented in this book—still leads this sort of life.

Here's the scoop on bowel activity: The vast majority of Americans move their bowels only a few times a week. That being the case, where the heck does all that built-up waste matter go? Well, it doesn't go anywhere! It remains tightly compacted in your bowels, normally in the sigmoid colon, sometimes in what is called the cecum, and sometimes in little sacs called diverticuli that are formed to hold solid waste products that accumulate.

That's right, all that gunk remains stored in your bowels until you finally clean it out—that is, unless your body functions properly and your bowels regularly move after every meal. (Ideally, a bowel movement will take place within sixty minutes after a meal.)

When this matter is allowed to remain in your system, health problems are imminent. Your bowels are forced to expand to store it, and your engorged bowels press against other internal organs in turn, thereby causing further health problems.

This solid waste matter builds up in the form of layers that are virtually "glued" to the walls of your digestive tract. The longer the waste is allowed to remain there, the more clogged the system becomes. In addition, this coating of dead material will slowly encrust the walls of your colon.

The problem is, for the rest of our lives we will be ingesting considerable amounts of environmental and digestive toxins (chemicals in our food, pollutants in the air, an occasional soft drink, toxins in our water supply, etc.) that we must regularly eliminate from our bodies. Unless we properly excrete this stuff, not only will our metabolic system suffer, but the overall state of our health will decline.

By doing a thorough cleansing of your system, you will enable your metabolism and your digestive system to make full use of the nutrients available in the foods you eat, so that you'll get more power from fewer calories. And therein lies the secret to permanent weight loss. However, before you can benefit from a cleanse, you must get your bowels working.

Here are a few simple techniques you can use to accomplish this; these are techniques that you'll be responsible for performing today.

The solution to buildup of solid waste

I strongly recommend that you cleanse your entire digestive tract on a weekly basis—or every other week at the very least. I showed you exactly how to do that in chapter 4: scraping away at the built-up matter and eventually flushing all of it away, thereby allowing your system to function as efficiently as possible. That process is very healthful, and it provides a great source of live enzymes and perfectly combined nutrients for your body and mind.

Right now, I want you to decide how often you're going to go through that cleansing process. Will you cleanse your system once a week? Every two weeks? Every Sunday? Only once in a blue moon? Be specific in your planning, and be sure to write it down or it won't get done.

Today's assignment

1. In an earlier chapter, we discussed the importance of consuming no less than one cup of water per day for every fourteen pounds of body weight. Figure out how much water that comes to for a person of your weight, and then find a nice-looking container that holds at least that much. Commit to filling that container with water each morning and then drinking the contents throughout the day, each and every day. Start drinking that much water today. More is better! In fact, you should consume a few extra glasses of water on days when you're going through the cleansing process.
2. Start the day (today) by mixing the juice of one lemon with a glass of plain, fresh (preferably distilled) water. Consume this at least ten to thirty minutes before you consume anything else.
3. Once the requisite time has elapsed, you may consume any fruit or vegetable juice, just as long as you juice it yourself—bottled or canned fruit juices are not allowed.
4. You may wish to make a broth by placing some fresh, organic vegetables in distilled water and cooking them over low heat, until the vegetables are soft.
5. Consume no fewer than three servings of fresh, raw, high-fiber vegetables (preferably organic) throughout the day, and have two or more servings of high-fiber fruits such as apples or figs as well.
6. The better the vegetables, the better the cleanse. Everyone has his or her favorites. List yours in your journal. But first, I want you to do some research on the health benefits of various vegetables. Find out which vegetables help certain ailments and which ones work best together. Get yourself one of the many good books that are available on vegetable juicing.
7. Now here's the kicker. We want to stimulate our colon muscles to evacuate any built-up matter that it may be harboring. To do this, we're going to use an herb that has many health benefits: cayenne. This herb helps to strengthen the blood and the internal organs, improves blood flow, and stimulates all the systems of the body,

from the brain to the digestive system. Today's goal will be to consume 1/4 teaspoonful of fresh cayenne powder in a bit of water or juice—and to repeat this every day. Once you get used to that serving size, gradually increase the amount to one full teaspoonful per day. Cayenne will stimulate and help strengthen your bowels, cleaning them out and making them strong again.

> Just a note of caution: cayenne is spicy hot, so you should notice a hot, tingling sensation when you consume it, but it's very good for your health—so much so that you shouldn't go for even a single day without drinking the prescribed cayenne solution. And try to avoid substituting the cayenne capsules found in health-food stores for the fresh cayenne powder that's called for. We want this very healthful herb to actually touch every inch of our digestive tract, stimulating the walls of our intestines as it moves through our system.

Lighting Your Metabolic Fire

The focus of this book has been threefold: to rev up your metabolic rate, to increase your fitness level, and to improve your physical and mental health. It's now time to *ignite the fire* by improving your food choices.

Day Three. On this day, day three, you're going to start your food program. As promised, I've included an example of what your diet could look like. Obviously, every person is different. Since it's impossible for me to sit across from you and create a diet that's specific to your individual body, this is about the best I can do.

Throughout this book, I've tried to educate you and change your way of thinking about food. Hopefully, you can make appropriate alterations to the example diet and adapt it to your particular needs. If I've been successful in imparting to you a general sense of what works and what doesn't, you should have enough information to determine the basic changes that need to be made. Now don't get me wrong. You will probably be somewhat confused—everyone is at first. Nevertheless, if you use the example diet I've provided, along with the techniques outlined in this text, I promise that you'll do fine.

Add the following eating program to the success you've already enjoyed on days one and two, and you'll be well on your way to making a tremendous shift in your metabolism, your appearance, and your destiny.

The example diet was designed for a woman who weighs approximately 150 pounds and wishes to attain a much leaner, healthier, more vibrant body. If you weigh more than 150 or are male, you will need to increase your intake of protein and vegetables. Women should consume an additional 50 calories for every 5 pounds of weight over 150. Men should add 500 calories (mainly from protein and vegetable sources) to the baseline calorie count, plus another 200 calories for every 25 pounds of weight over 175.

The baseline for phase one, diet #1 is 1868 calories, so a man who weighs 225 pounds at the start of this program would consume about 2768 calories on diet #1:

$$\begin{aligned} &\mathbf{1868 + 500 + \{200 \times [(225 - 175) \div 25]\}} \\ &\mathbf{= 2368 + \{200 \times [50 \div 25]\}} \\ &\mathbf{= 2368 + \{200 \times 2\}} \\ &\mathbf{= 2368 + 400} \\ &\mathbf{= 2768} \end{aligned}$$

A woman who weighs 175 at the start of the program would consume about 2118 calories on diet #1:

$$\begin{aligned} &\mathbf{1868 + \{50 \times [(175 - 150) \div 5]\}} \\ &\mathbf{= 1868 + \{50 \times [25 \div 5]\}} \\ &\mathbf{= 1868 + \{50 \times 5\}} \\ &\mathbf{= 1868 + 250} \\ &\mathbf{= 2118} \end{aligned}$$

Phase one of the dieting program is to be followed for (tentatively) a period of sixty to ninety days; it consists of three separate diets, each of which will draw you closer to your goal in its own way.

Phase two is a maintenance diet, one that will help you maintain your new, hard-earned physique. Once you graduate from phase one to phase two, be sure to follow diet #2 (as laid out in this book) for two days each week; on the remaining five days

Phase One, Diet #1

Meal	Food	Calories	Protein (g)	Carbs (g)	Fats (g)
0	1 cup warm water w/ 2 tbsp. lemon juice added				
1	2 servings of grits or cream of rice	200	4.4	44.0	0.8
	3 egg whites, large*	48	10.1	1.1	0.0
2	1 cup nonfat, sugar-free yogurt	70	13.2	4.3	0.0
	¼ cup Grape-Nuts *(optional)*	100	3.3	21.2	0.1
3	6 oz. turkey breast*	386	58.4	8.0	6.6
	1 mixed salad, large*	86	2.5	8.4	0.0
4	1 sweet potato, large*	236	2.4	48.8	0.4
	½ cup broccoli*	30	1.3	4.8	0.0
5	6 oz. chicken breast*	386	58.4	8.0	6.6
	1 mixed salad, large*	86	2.5	8.4	0.0
	½ cup brown rice*	240	8.0	52.0	2.0
Total		**1868**	**164.5**	**209.0**	**16.5**
Calories		**1868**	**790**	**836**	**149**
Percentage of Total Calories (%)		**100**	**42**	**45**	**8**

*See the diet notes that start on p. 187.

of the week, you should make a point of eating food that's generally considered healthful.

Although the diets we're talking about here were designed to be followed for longer than thirty days, your results will be dramatic—and will be realized in thirty days or less!—if you follow the entire MYM program put forth in this book. Remember, the diet itself is merely one piece of the overall success puzzle.

This dieting program was developed through use of an in-depth health history and an in-office consultation with each of my clients, with the intention of providing them with the nutrients needed to **burn any subcutaneous fat deposits, increase lean muscle strength (not size), increase energy level, and improve the digestive system.** To help clients achieve the desired results as quickly as possible, the three phase-one diets were used in conjunction with the example exercise program that's presented later in this chapter.

Diet #1 is to be strictly adhered to for a period of two days, then diet #2 for the next three days, and finally diet #3 for the last two days of a seven-day cycle, at which point the entire cycle is to be repeated. Alternating your diets like this is a powerful way to increase your metabolism. The two-day, three-day, two-day pattern presented in this chapter is designed to fully stimulate your metabolism, to maximum efficiency. If you feel as though you're burning too much fat too fast, however, you can use the following pattern instead: diet #1 for the first two days, then diet #2 for the next two days, and finally diet #3 for the last three days of a seven-day cycle, at which point this entire cycle is to be repeated. This cycling of nutrients and calories enables the metabolism to attain its peak fat-burning level.

One word of caution: water intake during a program like this cannot be allowed to fall below one gallon per day.

Diet #1 was designed to help strip fat and water from the area between the muscle and the skin.

Diet #2 is intended to deplete your muscles of both glycogen and water. Following this diet for three consecutive days will increase the rate at which your metabolism burns fat and decrease the sensitivity of your muscle cells to water, thereby causing them to release any stored water. Because of the lack of carbohydrates (in particular, sugars) consumed on these days, you may experience one or more of the following:

- Tendency to be more temperamental than usual
- Slightly greater-than-usual weight loss (due to loss of water)
- Increase in perspiration
- Craving for sweets
- Increase in urination

Phase One, Diet #2

Meal	Food	Calories	Protein (g)	Carbs (g)	Fats (g)
0	1 cup warm water w/ 2 tbsp. lemon juice added				
1	3–6 egg whites, large*	48	10.1	1.1	0.0
	2 rice cakes, plain*	70	1.5	16.0	0.0
2	6 oz. turkey breast*	386	58.4	8.0	6.6
	1 mixed salad, large*	86	2.5	8.4	0.0
3	3 slices fat-free American cheese	180	36.0	2.0	2.4
	5 fat-free crackers	50	2.1	11.2	0.0
4	3 oz. grilled meat*	156	25.4	0.0	5.9
	1 mixed salad, large*	86	2.5	8.4	0.0
Total		**1062**	**138.5**	**55.1**	**14.9**
Calories		**1062**	**665**	**220**	**134**
Percentage of Total Calories (%)		**100**	**63**	**21**	**13**

*See the diet notes that start on p. 187.

Please be advised that these are normal "withdrawal symptoms" that may occur as a result of the small quantity of sugar you're consuming. As stated earlier, this program was specifically designed to rid your body of such harmful things as sugar, toxins, and excess fat deposits. During the period when these undesirable substances are being eliminated (which usually occurs during the first fourteen days), you may consume a small piece of fruit (to deal with the effects of withdrawal from sugar) if you begin to feel lethargic or slightly dizzy.

Phase One, Diet #3

Meal	Food	Calories	Protein (g)	Carbs (g)	Fats (g)
0	1 cup warm water w/ 2 tbsp. lemon juice added				
1	1 serving of grits or cream of rice	100	2.2	22.0	0.4
	5 egg whites, large*	80	16.8	1.7	0.0
	spinach *(optional)*, in quantity desired*	—	—	—	—
2	1 6-oz. can water-packed tuna, drained*	180	36.0	2.0	2.4
	¼ cup brown rice*	120	4.0	26.0	1.0
3	6 oz. turkey breast*	386	58.4	8.0	6.6
	1 mixed salad, large*	86	2.5	8.4	0.0
4	6 oz. fish*	156	25.4	0.0	5.9
	1 mixed salad, large*	86	2.5	8.4	0.0
Total		**1194**	**147.8**	**76.5**	**16.3**
Calories		**1194**	**709**	**306**	**147**
Percentage of Total Calories (%)		**100**	**59**	**26**	**12**

*See the diet notes given below.

Diet notes

- If you are hungry or feel the need for additional food, you may increase your consumption of the protein sources (chicken, turkey, egg whites, tuna, and fish) at any of the meals for phase one during the first two weeks, but by day 15 you must be 100 percent on target with your food consumption.
- Either sliced or ground turkey (the 98% fat-free variety) may be substituted for chicken if you use it in the same quantity. Both chicken and turkey should be measured after cooking. Six ounces of meat is about the same size as two decks of playing cards.

- While on this diet, you are permitted to consume any type of fish *other than* carp, herring, mackerel, mullet, salmon, sardines, squid, and tuna steak.
- For purposes of this diet, the term *grilled meat* refers to any very lean red or white meat (beef, pork, turkey, or chicken). As long as you're on this program, be sure that before you consume *any* type of meat, you remove all the skin and visible fat prior to cooking.
- For purposes of this diet, the term *mixed salad* refers to any combination of raw, non-starchy vegetables (one that's devoid of starchy vegetables such as potatoes, avocados, and beans).
- Your may substitute a pure protein drink in place of chicken/turkey or eggs, provided you make the substitution according to the following formula: two scoops of protein powder mixed in water is equivalent to either three egg whites or 3 oz. of chicken or turkey. Be sure not to make this substitution at more than one meal on any given day. For purposes of this book, a pure protein drink is one which contains at least 40 grams of protein and less than 5 grams of carbohydrates in each serving.
- Fish or sushi/sashimi may be substituted for tuna or chicken in this phase: 3 oz. of sushi is equivalent to 3 oz. of chicken or 1/2 of a 6-oz. can of tuna.
- A medium, plain baked potato may be substituted for 1/2 cup of rice. If you make this substitution, be sure to remove the skin from the potato prior to eating it.
- Rice should be measured *prior* to cooking.
- Vegetable quantities should be measured *after* cooking.
- Candy that is both sugar free *and* sodium free may be eaten periodically throughout the day.
- For the first two weeks of the program, bagels, English muffins, and rice cakes can be considered interchangeable as long as you substitute one of them for another according to the following formula: two rice cakes is equivalent to either one medium bagel or one whole English muffin. You should be aware of the possibility that this substitution will slightly retard your weight loss.

- When preparing your meals, avoid using any butter, margarine, oil, mayonnaise, prepared sauces, or salt. In place of these items, you may substitute any herb or herbal product (no salt or fat), and—for the first two weeks ONLY—you may use fat-free salad dressing, fat-free butter (*promise*), or fat-free mayonnaise (but there is a limit of one tablespoon per meal, total, for these last three ingredients).
- You may experience an increase in urination and/or defecation during this phase of the program. This is due, in part, to the delicate cleansing effect that this particular combination of foods has on your digestive system, and in part to an increase in your metabolic rate.
- At some point during the first two weeks of this phase, you may experience a slight increase in intestinal gas. This is normal; it's caused by the elimination of previously built-up matter within your system. The release of this matter is a mandatory step toward a fully functioning digestive system.

Today's assignment

1. Spend time making slight modifications to the three example diets given above for phase one. Show them to your physician or your health-care professional if you wish, and then get started.
2. That's it. You have enough on your plate for today. Just keep to the diets, make some notes in your journal, and commit to following this new way of eating for at least the next sixty to ninety days.

STOP HERE!

Don't go any further unless you've completed every part of each of the previous assignments. This is not a race. It's a training process for your metabolism, and it must be undertaken in a systematic way. Each day, do your exercises in full, make notes in your personal journal, and continue implementing and improving that day's exercises for a period of thirty days (or as otherwise indicated). As you get to each of the upcoming days (days four through seven), add that new day's activities to your ongoing exercises from all the days prior to it.

How to Add Octane to Your Cardiovascular Training

Congratulations! You're one of a relatively small contingent of readers who have made it this far. Most people put the book down after the previous section. What your persistence demonstrates is that you're one of those in that top 10 percent of the population who truly want to improve their health and their appearance—and you will succeed! Now let's maximize your metabolism by training your cardiovascular system.

Day Four. Your metabolic fitness includes both aerobic and strength-training elements that work together to produce total metabolic health. You simply cannot have the whole package without including physical training and a systematic, healthful diet.

As you learned previously, aerobic (cardiovascular) exercises are those that burn huge amounts of oxygen. Do you remember what they are? Here are a few examples:

running

jogging

aerobics classes

spinning® classes

power walking

indoor rock climbing

Exercises such as these place heavy demands on your heart and lungs; they are excellent methods for promoting cardiovascular fitness. Cardiovascular exercise is also known to

- Burn calories and help regulate appetite
- Lift your mood
- Relieve depression, boredom, fatigue, and stress

Regardless of the program you choose, I recommend that your entire exercise program include the following five elements:

1. Aerobic warm-up
2. Minor stretching
3. Aerobic and strength conditioning
4. Aerobic cool-down
5. Final, more-detailed stretching

Now not everyone will have the time for all five of these activities, but you should never miss your warm-up, or the actual aerobic and strength-training session, or your cool-down. The stretching is very helpful, but for purposes of this program the stretching is slightly less important than the cardiovascular part. However, you should not let more than thirty days go by without including a stretching component in your exercise routine.

The warm-up elevates the core temperature of your muscles, increases the pulse rate and blood flow throughout your body, and gets your body ready for exercise. Stretching prepares the body for exercise by improving the elasticity of the muscles, which helps to prevent injury. The aerobic exercise you choose should be performed within your target heart range (THR). The simplest way to determine your THR is the following formula, which gives lower and upper bounds on the heart rate you should aim for:

(220 minus your age) multiplied by 0.70 = your lower bound

(220 minus your age) multiplied by 0.80 = your upper bound

Monitor your heart rate by using a heart-rate monitor strapped to your chest (this can be purchased for around $75 in any fitness store). Be sure to keep your heart rate within your target heart range (THR) during your entire period of aerobic exercise (that is, keep it between the lower and upper bounds given by the above formula).

The cool-down is really just the opposite of the warm-up. The rate at which you exercise (and your heart rate) should slowly decrease during the cool-down, thereby allowing your body to eliminate harmful lactates and return to a normal temperature.

Now set some short-term goals, say weekly, for the amount of time you will spend on the actual aerobic-conditioning phase of your exercise routine. If you can perform only ten minutes' worth of moderate cardiovascular exercise at this point, then setting a goal of working up to a thirty-minute exercise period within the next seven days is neither attainable nor safe. **Pushing yourself too hard will not increase your metabolism. What is needed for an increase in metabolism is persistent training (that is, being sure not to miss your scheduled training sessions).** Increasing the length of your cardio session by, let's say, five minutes on every third workout is a great goal—one that will constantly increase your metabolic rate—but stop increasing the length of your cardio workouts once you get up to sixty minutes.

As for the intensity of each of your training sessions, remember to monitor your heart rate so that you will always be in the correct fat-burning, metabolic-enhancing range. Whatever your level of aerobic/cardiovascular activity, select and *write out* your goals, then focus wholeheartedly on achieving those goals. And do it now.

Today's assignment

1. Write out your cardiovascular goals (for example, to do some form of aerobic conditioning four times each week, for thirty minutes each time).
2. Commit to keeping to the following schedule for the next thirty days:
    a. Five minutes of a general warm-up
    b. Five minutes of light stretching
    c. At least thirty minutes of aerobic conditioning (we'll add your strength training tomorrow, on day five)
    d. Ten minutes of a general cool-down
    e. Ten minutes of light stretching
3. **Never set a schedule without actually starting to follow it that very day!** Start and complete your first aerobic session according to the schedule laid out above.
4. Write out a schedule of the exact times at which you will train each day for the next few days. In fact, you should get into the habit of writing out the next day's schedule each night before you go to bed.

This is a good place to make a side note regarding your journal entries. You should be writing out your goals on a regular basis, either daily or weekly. The more you write and re-write your goals, the more ingrained in your subconscious they will become. So make this a regular practice, and never miss a journal entry.

Building Dense, Well-Toned Muscles

The other half of the fitness equation is the development of muscle strength and endurance, what we'll call strength training. Today, day five, you'll begin to accelerate your progress tenfold, by incorporating strength training into your program.

Day Five. Muscle endurance is the ability of muscles to apply a sub-maximal force repeatedly or to be exercised over an extended period of time. Here are some common means of building muscle endurance:

free weights

exercise machines

push-ups, sit-ups, chin-ups

Of these three, my favorite is the use of free weights. No matter what your goals are, free weights give you greater control over your destiny. In the absence of free weights (dumbbells or barbells), you can resort to push-ups, sit-ups, etc.; however, your progress will be slower and harder to track.

One of the principal benefits of muscle conditioning is that muscles serve as the body's motor, burning most of the energy it produces. Losing muscle density while continuing to take in the same amount of energy in the form of food has the undesirable outcome of causing you to put on weight in the form of fat.

When we reach our thirties, we begin to lose muscle mass, for a myriad of reasons. As we age, our basal metabolic rate decreases by about one-half of one percent per year. Thus, our overall metabolic rate will naturally start slowing as we get older *unless we can increase our muscle density*. The way we do this in the *Maximize Your Metabolism* program is through strength training.

Keep in mind that every pound of muscle burns approximately fifty calories per day. Thus, for every pound of muscle you gain, you can eat fifty additional calories' worth of food each day without gaining weight in the form of fat. Better yet, make your diet a bit more healthful and gain a few pounds of muscle density, and then see what happens. What you will undoubtedly find is that you'll have a rapid drop in body fat on account of your heightened metabolism! Obviously, the opposite is also true. Lose a pound of muscle mass (and you'll lose a lot of muscle mass if you don't exercise regularly and properly), and you'll have to cut back on your food intake by fifty or more calories a day in order to avoid gaining weight.

Traditionally, weight-loss science has taught that optimum metabolism can be achieved by balancing the sources of energy. In short, what goes in must equal what goes out. If the energy equivalent of the food you eat is more than the energy you burn, you'll *gain* weight. If you burn more energy than the equivalent of what you ingest in the way of food, you'll *lose* weight.

However, that's not the whole story. There is also an adaptive effect of dieting: the greater the number of times you restrict your calories for a prolonged period of time, the slower your metabolism becomes. The slower your metabolism, the more calories your body will store as body fat the next time you eat.

The best way to combat this natural tendency to conserve energy is to reset your metabolic rate with a comprehensive program of strength training and aerobic activity. A balanced fitness program will help you make permanent weight loss a part of your life.

It's far more efficient to use exercise as a metabolic-boosting and fat-burning strategy for losing weight than it is to count on diet alone. In fact, we tend to burn off calories both *during* and *after* exercise. Strength-building exercises fire up our caloric "furnace" and raise our resting metabolic rate.

Weight training has the added effect of breaking down muscle tissue. In reality, you *injure* your muscle tissue when you lift weights, but if you rest the affected muscles and supply them with proper nutrients, they'll automatically seek to protect themselves from further injury by becoming stronger and more responsive. This may sound like a harsh, masochistic approach to fitness, but it's totally natural and very good for your health.

Your body adapts to the stress of weight training by repairing the injured muscle tissue and then stimulating growth of new muscle tissue in order to overcome the additional workload. In essence, your muscles become stronger and denser to overcome the added stress.

Now don't be alarmed. I know what you're thinking: "It sounds as if I have to become a bodybuilder or at least gain tons in the way of muscular size." That's not what muscle density means. We discussed this earlier, but I feel compelled to review it now. Muscle *density* refers to the strength, health, and tightness of your muscles, while muscle *size* refers to their volume. You can greatly increase your muscle density without increasing your muscle size! If your goal is to gain in muscular size, slight modifications can be made to this program to accomplish that goal, but this book is focused on gaining in muscle density, not size.

Since strength-building exercises exert stresses on your muscles, they require an increased flow of blood in order to carry on their restorative and strengthening processes. When blood is forced into your muscles during your weightlifting program, it helps speed up the repair process in your muscle tissues. As they rebuild themselves, they become denser and stronger than they were before. That's why it is so important for you to follow your strength-training regimen to the letter, and to combine that program with a good diet and proper rest.

Your strength-training routine

Always start out with an easy strength-training regimen, perhaps with a one-set, ten-rep program of eight to ten different exercises, two or three times a week.

Your normal routine might include a warm-up, followed by some squats, and then some pull-downs, bench presses, bicep curls, tricep push-downs, side laterals, incline sit-ups (or leg lifts), and finally a cardio regimen. Make sure you do your exercises in the proper order.

Typically, your personal trainer (if you're lucky enough to have a good one) will recommend starting with a larger muscle group and working your way down to a smaller one. Always train your muscle groups in an organized, systematic fashion, and complete all the sets for each exercise (if you're doing more than one) before going on to another exercise. Once you establish a particular order in which to work your muscles, stick to that order (unless otherwise noted by your trainer) for thirty days before modifying it and adding variety.

Exercise sets

Just a refresher: A *rep* (short for "repetition") is a single performance of one particular weight-lifting or exercise movement. A *set* consists of the sum total of all the times that you engage in a particular movement in succession before taking a rest. The best exercise system for increasing your metabolism is to do three to four sets of eight to twelve reps each. In this system, you should choose a weight that can be lifted ONLY eight to twelve times (meaning that you are actually incapable of lifting the weight one more time after you reach the eighth or twelfth rep, respectively). Then you should repeat the sequence two or three more times (that is, do two or three more *sets*), allowing just enough rest in between sets for you to recover. Normally, your rest time between sets will be about thirty seconds.

The secret of progressive resistance

As muscles adapt to a particular level of resistance (for example, the amount of weight you lift or the amount of rest time between sets), you should gradually increase your resistance, either by increasing the amount of weight you lift or decreasing your rest period between sets. This must occur if you are to continue to reap the benefits of the exercise in the form of denser, stronger muscles and an ever-increasing metabolism caused by those denser muscles. If you don't increase your resistance from time to time, your program will still be beneficial, but you probably won't develop the muscular density that you have set as your goal.

Progressively increasing your resistance is your key to muscle density and metabolic enhancement through anaerobic (weight) training. The progression principle requires that as soon as the weight you are lifting is no longer causing sufficient stress on your muscles, you must either increase your resistance or decrease your rest time between sets. That way, you'll ensure that the workout continues to be a challenge for you.

Always exercise in proper form. The key to realizing the maximum metabolic benefit through weight training is found not in just *doing* an exercise—regardless of style or form—but in doing it *correctly*, so that you'll get the most out of every exercise you do.

Your exercising motions should be clean and fluid, and directly in line with the proper axis of the muscle being worked. If you can possibly help it, you shouldn't allow your line of exercise motion to stray. Instruction in how to perform any given exercise correctly can be obtained from a fitness coach or a personal trainer at a good health club.

In addition to lifting *form*, lifting *speed* is an important element that has a major effect on the flow of blood to your target muscles. And while you might think better results are to be realized from lifting weights at a faster pace, the opposite is actually true. Although fast lifting creates a certain momentum, it doesn't promote optimal blood flow to the muscle, so it pays to slow down a bit.

Always listen to your body. If your body tells you there's something that isn't right, then stop the exercise immediately and rest for a few days before attempting that particular exercise again. But continue with all other aspects of your training and diet.

The next thirty days

Here you are! The next thirty days will change your life, forever! Have you been completing your daily activities and exercises so far? If not, stop here and make sure you're on target up to this point. Then once you are, you may proceed.

The exercise routine presented in the table below is a sample of one that I used with several clients of mine who had made tremendous progress and surpassed their goals. I've included it here, not necessarily for you to follow but so that you can see what a well-structured routine looks like. Study it and then create your own routine, using the one given here as a skeleton to build upon and personalize for your particular level of experience.

The clients who used this routine had already had a fair amount of experience in exercising, and they knew all about proper form for each of the exercises listed in the table. What they did not know was how to put their knowledge to use to achieve the results they wanted. Only after years of trial and error did they decide to consult me. This exercise routine, which I assigned to them, brought not only the kinds of results they sought but many more besides.

Today's assignment

1. Review the exercise routine that's laid out in the following table and make any modifications you see fit, but keep the general structure, such as the order of the exercises. You may even want to keep the exercises themselves.
2. Before your first workout, write out a clear and concise goal for what you want to achieve in the next thirty days of training. Then commit to never missing a workout. You might wish to use one of my favorite slogans: "miss your favorite television show, but never miss one of your training sessions."
3. Have fun. This is not work. This is the way you scientifically and systematically reach your goals. The process can be fun, but you must force yourself to be persistent.

MYM *(Maximize Your Metabolism)* Workout*

	Days 1 to 30			**Days 31 to 60**		
Exercise	**Sets**	**Reps**	**Rest (sec.)**	**Sets**	**Reps**	**Rest (sec.)**
Legs						
Squats	3	10–15	30–45	3	8–10	20–30
Stiff-leg deadlifts	3	10–15	30–45	3	8–10	20–30
Lunges	0	—	—	3	8–10	20–30
Back						
One-arm row	3	10–15	30–45	3	8–10	20–30
Pull-downs	0	—	—	3	8–10	20–30
Chest						
Incline bench	3	10–15	30–45	3	8–10	20–30
Flat flies	0	—	—	3	8–10	20–30
Shoulders						
Upright row	3	10–15	30–45	3	10–12	20–30
Bent lateral	0	—	—	3	10–12	20–30
Biceps						
Alternating D-bell curls	3	15–20	30–45	3	8–12	20–30
Concentrating curls	0	—	—	3	8–10	20–30
Triceps						
Tricep kick-backs	3	10–15	30–45	3	8–10	20–30
Overhead extensions	0	—	—	3	8–12	20–30
Abdominals						
Lying leg lift	2	10–15	15	2	20–25	15
Reverse crunches	1	10	0	1	20	0
Crunches	1	15	0	1	25	0
Parallel crunches	1	10	0	1	10	0

*Begin each workout with ten minutes of light aerobics, and end it with twenty to forty-five minutes of the same.

Day Six. We've already talked about the importance of a personal journal in helping you keep your eye on what's going on in your program. But now we're going to explain precisely how to build your goals by use of your journal. In the process of doing that, we'll be planning your physical destiny.

I once heard a professional speaker named Zig Ziglar give an explanation of the importance of goals. I have used his approach to achieving goals many times, and I'd like to share it with you now.

Ziglar told of a world-famous archer who could hit the bull's-eye using a bow and arrow nearly every time he attempted it. He went on to say that he could teach anyone to be more accurate with a bow and arrow, and even to hit the target more often on average—and closer to the center of the bull's-eye—than that expert archer could. The way Zig proposed to do this was to blindfold the archer, spin him around several times, and then give him no clue as to where the target was.

That may sound silly at first. How could this world-renowned archer possibly hit a target if he were blindfolded and dizzy? But it very astutely illustrates my point about setting goals: **You cannot hit a goal you do not have.**

Setting goals is a vital part of many of our accomplishments. In fact, I'd be willing to bet that you've never achieved anything worthwhile in life without first having set the attainment of that particular milestone as a goal. You may not have been aware that you were setting a goal. You may not have actually gotten your goal down on paper. You may not even have thought of it as a goal, but you did desire to attain it, and so you subconsciously set that goal in your mind.

You may be able to speed up the achievement of your goals by following the formula given below, but only if you are persistent in your efforts.

Your formula for success

1. Set a goal for yourself.
2. Become highly passionate about attaining this goal.
3. Clearly write out your goal.
4. Write out a detailed "plan of action," with monthly, weekly, and daily steps, and be persistent in following your plan.
5. About thirty times each day, think about how great it will

be to have achieved this goal—in essence, become *obsessed* with its attainment.

6. Stay on top of your plan of action, and if you notice that it isn't working, study the situation and then make changes to your plan to help improve upon it.

Today's assignment

1. Complete the exercise on Crystallizing Your Focus found in the chapter on desire (chapter 3), and then have your number-one goal in front of you when you set out to do today's exercises.
2. No goal can be properly set or achieved without a sufficiently strong desire for its attainment. Write out, in a special place in the front of your journal, exactly why you desire to achieve your goal. If you are really on track, you'll get a bit emotional about it. If you don't get emotional about your goal, then it's not the right goal for you, and you probably won't have enough desire to be persistent in trying to achieve it.
3. Write out a clear description of your goal. As you do this, you can follow an approach that's similar to what you used in doing step #2 of today's assignment, but you need to chisel down the description of your goal to a powerful two- to three-sentence statement that gets you focused and jazzed up just by reading it.
4. Neatly rewrite the description of your goal at the top of a clean page in your journal. A line or two below that, write the words "Plan of Action." Now get *very* detailed, and write a list of *everything* you need to do to reach your goal. Finally, write out exactly how you will achieve each of these "sub-goals."
5. As I said before, you need to be flexible in your approach. Modify your plan if you figure that by modifying it you'll be likely to reach your goal even sooner. But be careful: Study your plan and your potential modification carefully. Don't rush into any changes to your plan. If you find yourself making frequent or rushed changes, then you know you're just procrastinating—and ultimately setting yourself up for failure.

At this point, I'd like to include a brief discussion on being flexible. I prefer to illustrate my view of flexibility like this: Picture a field with two trees in it, one of them large, about fifty feet tall, and strong looking; the other still young, only about ten feet tall, and relatively thin. If only one of these trees survives in a major windstorm, it won't be the larger one, the one that refused to bend in the wind. The tree that will survive is the younger, smaller one, because it was flexible and let the wind bend it temporarily. Now, don't get me wrong; I am very adamant about holding to my vision and my goals. But the approach I take to reaching my goals, and the approach you take to reaching yours, must be filled with desire, must be written out clearly, and must be flexible enough to be modified if necessary.

6. One additional element that's absolutely essential in setting goals is a deadline. None of your goals will be reached on time if you have no deadlines! Whenever you set a deadline for yourself, be sure that it's reasonable and attainable, but one that scares you a bit as well!

Day Seven. This is your day for rest and play. As you know, all work and no play makes Jack (and Jill) just as dull as can be. And though you should reward yourself once in a while, you're on a mission right now and you want to keep up the momentum for the next thirty days without veering off course—not even once.

The resting and playing I'm referring to here are to be physical in nature. This is your chance to rest your body and exercise your mind.

Yes, I know, you think you've been exercising your mind the whole time you've been reading this book and doing the exercises laid out herein. But now we're going to put your mind through mental boot camp. We're going to crank up the volume on your desire to attain your goal. And most importantly, we're going to set up a "success mindset" for you.

You may recall that a few chapters back I told you that when you train with weights, rather than just doing aerobic exercises, your body responds by burning calories during your exercise routine as well as for a long time after you're finished exercising for the day. I used the example of burning calories (body fat) while you sleep.

Well, now we're going to program your mind so that it's focused on achieving your goal even when you're focused on your normal daily activities. Let's think of this process as one of training your mind so well *now* that you can run it on autopilot *later*. Even when you're not focused on achieving your goal, your mind will be drawing it into your life!

Okay. Enough explanation. This is a hard-core, "just-do-it" kind of exercise, so let's move on to the daily assignment.

Today's assignment

1. You have already written a really good affirmation (the two- to three-sentence statement of your achieving your goal). Now take that affirmation, and read it out loud at least a hundred times today. Do this in a place where no one can hear or see you! In fact, don't tell anyone about this exercise, or even that you *have* a goal. *Let others see the results in full before you let them in on the existence of your goal or how you have accomplished it.* Take several breaks from your normal day today, and, with great excitement, repeat your success statement ten to twenty times. When you do this, make sure you're visualizing yourself as having already achieved your goal.

   This is very important, so I'll say it again: when you repeat your success statement, make sure you are highly emotional about it (get excited) and be sure to visualize yourself as having already achieved your goal (see yourself in the shape you're aiming for—and see yourself being congratulated by others).

2. Even when you're not repeating your success statement, stay focused on the mental picture you have of yourself having already achieved your goal. At least four times today, take five to ten minutes to sit quietly in a room where you won't be disturbed; first relax, and then clearly visualize yourself having already achieved your goal. See the colors, hear the compliments of others, feel the clothes you have on, feel how great your new body feels. Get as many of your senses involved as you can. I know this will take time out of your day, but it will make a *dramatic* impact on the speed with which you reach your goal. And

the faster you reach your physical goal, the faster you can become more successful in all other areas of your life. Remember, not being in top shape holds you back in every aspect of your life. You may not understand that now, and that's OK. **Just take it on faith that once you've gotten into top shape physically, it will be a lot easier to achieve all your other goals—financial goals, relationship and family goals, business goals, etc.**

3. At the end of your day, while lying in bed, repeat your success statement to yourself, again visualizing yourself as having achieved your goal (this time in a relaxed state of mind—don't get excited or emotional). Do this over and over until you fall asleep. Make this the last thing you think about as you drift off. This will help to deeply root your affirmation in your subconscious mind.

That's it! You've done it!

You've completed the most powerful Seven Days of Training that you could ever come across. And you've done it all on your own!

Actually, you aren't quite finished yet! Remember that you are to use what you learned in this book (about yourself and about fitness) to continue these activities for a period of at least thirty days. Don't stop doing any of the activities you've been engaged in during the past seven days. Indeed, don't stop doing anything you've learned, regardless of where it's presented in this book.

The exercises prescribed for this seven-day period were designed to simply get the ball rolling. It's now your responsibility to keep it rolling. Your degree of success will be determined by the extent to which you keep moving forward, daily, in each of the areas we've discussed. Whenever you find that you aren't progressing fast enough or that you aren't heading in the right direction, just review what was presented here and figure out what aspect of this program you've become slack on. If you get to the point of needing an extra kick in the rear end, redo the entire last chapter. If there's one particular exercise in this chapter that you don't feel like doing, that's almost surely the one that's holding you back!

I have successfully used the information in this book with thousands of participants at my health clubs. *I know it works.* I know it will work for you if you follow it faithfully.

Good luck, and please keep in touch. My office is filled with letters from successful clients, and I would truly love to have a letter from you describing your success. In fact, I would like you to make that one of your goals. In thirty days, write me a short letter and let me know how you used this material to reach your goal. You might even include before-and-after pictures. If you do, I'll send you a Certificate of Completion and a small gift.

And remember this: I respect you, and I'm very proud of you for having read this entire book and gone through this program. I know what it takes to maximize your metabolism, and I know that these last seven days have been hectic for you, but keep in mind that there are lots of people out there who—like me—definitely want to see you succeed. And you're not alone in this; I'll always do my best to answer your health and fitness questions.

Here's to your health!

****

Be sure to visit me online at:
www.MaximizeYourMetabolism.com

Send your health and fitness questions to:
Questions@MaximizeYourMetabolism.com

Send your success stories to us at:
SuccessStories@MaximizeYourMetabolism.com

For a complete list of books, seminars, e-classes, audio programs, and newsletters written by Christopher Guerriero, please e-mail us at:
Courses@MaximizeYourMetabolism.com

FREE ONLINE CONSULTING

OFFER VALID ONLY FOR THE OWNER OF THIS BOOK

For more than fourteen years now, my goal has been to help the greatest number of people possible achieve their physical goals. Through seminars, e-classes, personal coaching, cassettes/CD's, newsletters, and books like this one, I'm happy to say that I've helped many thousands of people just like you attain the body they've always wanted - but previously thought was out of reach.

When I personally work with someone - which I rarely do any longer because of time constraints - my normal fee is $250 per hour.

For reading this whole book and following all the exercises laid out herein, I'm going to gift you with a block of my time. Enough time to answer any three e-questions that you have regarding the material in this book.

I've even created a special account for you to send in your questions. It's a private account that no-one will have access to except for me and the person who filters my e-mail.

To use this FREE ONLINE COACHING, simply send your three key questions to:

3FREE@MaximizeYourMetabolism.com

When preparing your questions, please include any pertinent information like your age, past fitness and dieting experience, current workout regimen, physical limitation, etc.

Bibliography

Chapter 2. The Magic of Beliefs, Values, Goals, and Persistence

Goal Setting

Baron, P., and Watters, R.G. (1981). Effects of goal-setting and of goal levels on weight loss induced by self-monitoring of caloric intake. *Canadian Journal of Behavioural Science*, 13(2):161–170.

Geis, J.A., and Klein, H.A. (1990). The relationship of life satisfaction to life change among the elderly. *Journal of Genetic Psychology*, 151(2):269–271.

Madsen, J., Sallis, J.F., Patterson, T., Rupp, J., Senn, K., Atkins, C., and Nader, P.R. (1989). The validity of self-monitoring of diet and exercise in a family-based health behavior change program. Presented at the 10th Annual Meeting of the Society of Behavioral Medicine, San Francisco, CA.

Chapter 8. Metabolic Superchargers That Work

Androstenedione

King, D.S., Sharp, R.L., Vukovich, M.D., Brown, G.A., Reifenrath, T.A., Uhl, N.L., and Parsons, K.A. (1999). Effect of oral androstenedione on serum testosterone and adaptations to resistance training in young men: a randomized controlled trial. *Journal of the American Medical Association*, 281(21):2020–2028.

Leder, B.Z., Longcope, C., Catlin, D.H., Ahrens, B., Schoenfeld, D.A., and Finkelstein, J.S. (2000). Oral androstenedione administration and serum testosterone concentrations in young men. *Journal of the American Medical Association*, 283(6):779–782.

Carnitine

Angelini, C., Vergani, L., Costa, L., Martinuzzi, A., Dunner, E., Marescotti, C., and Nasadini, R. (1986). Use of carnitine in exercise physiology. *Advances in Clinical Enzymology*, 4:103.

Chromium

Anderson, R.A., Polansky, M.M., Bryden, N.A., Roginski, E.E., Mertz, W., and Glinsmann, W. (1983). Chromium supplementation of human subjects: effects on glucose, insulin, and lipid variables. *Metabolism*, 32(9):894–899.

Anderson, R.A., Chromium as an essential nutrient for humans (1997). *Regulatory Toxicology and Pharmacology*, 26(1):S35–S41.

Ephedrine

Astrup, A., Breum, L., and Toubro, S. (1995). Pharmacological and clinical studies of ephedrine and other thermogenic agonists. *Obesity Research*, 3(Suppl. 4):537S–540S. Review.

Chapter 11. Oxygen Creates Movement Before Movement Creates Oxygen

Proper Breathing

Freedman, R.R., and Woodward, S. (1992). Behavioral treatment of menopausal hot flushes: evaluation by ambulatory monitoring. *American Journal of Obstetrics and Gynecology*, 167(2):436–439.

Grossman, E., Grossman, A., Schein, M.H., Zimlichman, R., and Gavish, B. (2001). Breathing-control lowers blood pressure. *Journal of Human Hypertension*, 15(4):263–269.

Chapter 12. Mastering Your Emotions and Your State of Mind

Endorphins: The Body's Natural Stress Relievers

Kolotkin, R.L., Head, S., Hamilton, M., and Tse, C.K. (1995). Assessing impact of weight on quality of life. *Obesity Research*, 3(1):49–56.

Chapter 13. Cut Years off of Your Efforts

Active Support

Black, D.R., Gleser, L.J., and Kooyers, K.J. (1990). A meta-analytic evaluation of couples weight-loss programs. *Health Psychology*, 9(3):330–347.

Lassner, J.B. (1991). Does social support aid in weight loss and smoking interventions? Reply from a family systems perspective. *Annals of Behavioral Medicine*, 13(2):66–72.

Books That Offer Models

Hill, N. (1990). *Think and Grow Rich.* Ballantine Books, New York, NY.

Maltz, M. (1970). *Psycho-Cybernetics.* Pocket Books/Simon & Schuster, New York, NY.

Chapter 16. Getting Yourself to Exercise Regularly

Why We Fade

Godin, G., Valois, P., Shephard, R.J., and Desharnais, R. (1987). Prediction of leisure-time exercise behavior: a path analysis (LISREL V) model. *Journal of Behavioral Medicine*, 10(2):145–158.

Shephard, R.J. (1995). Factors influencing the exercise behavior of patients. *Sports Medicine*, 2(5):348–366.

Chapter 17. Take Action: Your Motivational Challenge

Laser Visualization and Modeling

Ziglar, Z. (1998). *Success for Dummies*. John Wiley & Sons, New York, NY.

The Decision Is Now Yours

Kiefer, M.M. (1995). *The Powermind System: Twelve Lessons on the Psychology of Success*. Kiefer Enterprises International Press, Minnesota.

Index